Biosocialities, Genetics and the Social Sciences

T0173950

Investigations into the genetic make-up of humans have transformed the way we think about ourselves and the world around us. This not only affects the way we think about health and disease, but it also impacts on our ideas about what it is to be human. *Biosocialities, Genetics and the Social Sciences* explores the social, cultural and economic transformations that result from innovations in genomic knowledge and technology.

This pioneering collection uses Paul Rabinow's concept of biosociality to chart the shifts in social relations and in ideas about nature, biology and identity brought about by developments in biomedicine. Based on new empirical research, it contains chapters on genomic research into embryonic stem cell therapy, breast cancer, autism, Parkinson's and IVF treatment, as well as on the expectations and education surrounding genomic research.

Biosocialities, Genetics and the Social Sciences covers four main themes:

- Novel modes of identity and identification, such as genetic citizenship.
- The role of institutions, ranging from disease advocacy organisations and voluntary organisations to the state.
- The production of biological knowledge, novel life-forms, and technologies.
- The generation of wealth and commercial interests in biology.

Including an afterword by Paul Rabinow and case studies focusing on the UK, the US, Canada, Germany, India and Israel, this book will be of interest to students and researchers of the new genetics and the social sciences – particularly medical sociologists, medical anthropologists and those involved with science and technology studies.

Sahra Gibbon is currently undertaking a Wellcome Trust fellowship at University College London, UK.

Carlos Novas is a Wellcome Trust funded Postdoctoral Fellow at the BIOS Centre, London School of Economics, UK.

Biosocialities, Genetics and the Social Sciences

Making biologies and identities

Edited by
Sahra Gibbon and Carlos Novas

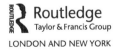

Routledge
Taylor & Francis Group

LONDON AND NEW YORK

First published 2008
by Routledge
2 Park Square, Milton Park, Abingdon, Oxon OX14 4RN

Simultaneously published in the USA and Canada
by Routledge
711 Third Avenue, New York, NY 10017

Routledge is an imprint of the Taylor & Francis Group, an informa business

© 2008 Selection and editorial matter, Sahra Gibbon and Carlos Novas;
individual chapters, the contributors

Typeset in Times New Roman by
HWA Text and Data Management, Tunbridge Wells

British Library Cataloguing in Publication Data
A catalogue record for this book is available from the British Library

Library of Congress Cataloging-in-Publication Data
A catalog record for this book has been requested

ISBN10: 0–415–40137–2 (hbk)
ISBN10: 0–415–40138–0 (pbk)
ISBN10: 0–203–94594–8 (ebk)

ISBN13: 978–0–415–40137–1 (hbk)
ISBN13: 978–0–415–40138–8 (pbk)
ISBN13: 978–0–203–94594–0 (ebk)

Contents

Contributors

Aditya Bharadwaj is a lecturer at the School of Social and Political Studies, University of Edinburgh. His principal research interest is in the area of new reproductive, genetic and stem cell biotechnologies and their rapid spread in diverse global locales ranging from South Asia to the United Kingdom. His research interests lie at an interface between cultural and biomedical dimensions of assisted reproduction in India. His past research has examined issues surrounding gender and reproductive health care with special reference to medically mediated childbirth, food and nutrition and immunisation. His recently concluded research, funded by ESRC's Innovative Health Technologies Programme, was located in South Wales. The research explains the consequences of population screening for genetic disorders based on the case of haemochromatosis.

Sahra Gibbon is a Post-Doctoral Research Fellow in the Department of Anthropology at University College London. She has a longstanding interest in the social and cultural dimenions of developments in genomics and the dynamic interface between differently constituted sciences and publics. She teaches on a range of courses focusing on the anthropology of medicine, science and technology.

Margaret Lock is Marjorie Bronfman Professor in Social Studies in Medicine, and is affiliated with the Department of Social Studies of Medicine and the Department of Anthropology at McGill University. She is a Fellow of the Royal Society of Canada and an Officier de l'Ordre National du Québec. Lock was awarded the Prix Du Québec, domaine Sciences Humaines in 1997 and in the same year the Wellcome Medal of the Royal Anthropological Society of Great Britain. In 2002 she received the Canada Council for the Arts Molson Prize, in 2005 the Canada Council for the Arts Killam Prize, and in the same year she was awarded a Trudeau Fellowship. Among her prize-winning monographs is *Twice Dead: Organ Transplants and the Reinvention of Death.* Her current research deals with the circulation of post-genomic knowledge among basic scientists, clinics, families, and society at large, with particular emphasis on a re-conceptualization of Alzheimer's disease.

Michal Nahman is a lecturer in the Sociology Department at Lancaster University. Her research focuses on the study of biomedicine and science as they relate to gender, nationalism, race and sexuality. She is currently working on a book titled *Israeli Extractions: An Ethnographic Study of Ova Donation and National Imaginaries.* This monograph deals with the politics of borders and bodies as they emerge through technoscientific discursive practices of extraction, exchange and implantation of human ova between differently situated women. As the research for this project was conducted during the second *Intifada*, and amid a rising fear of the 'demographic threat' of Palestinians to the Israeli state's existence, the book's theorizing of nationalism and identity is inevitably shaped by this context.

Carlos Novas is a Wellcome Trust Postdoctoral Fellow at the BIOS Centre for the Study of Bioscience, Biomedicine, Biotechnology and Society, London School of Economics. He is currently working on a project titled: 'The political economy of hope: private enterprise, patients' groups and the production of values in the contemporary life sciences'. This project aims to explore the values and ethical principles that underpin and are promoted by biotechnology firms and patients' organizations as they invest in and conduct genetic research. He has recently been appointed as an Assistant Professor at Carleton University, where he will begin teaching in September 2007.

Paul Rabinow is Professor of Anthropology at the University of California at Berkeley. A recent book is *Marking Time: On the Anthropology of the Contemporary* (2007). He is director of the Collaboratory for the Anthropology of the Contemporary (www.anthropos-lab.net). His current research concerns synthetic biology.

Elizabeth F.S. Roberts is a medical anthropologist and assistant research scientist at the Institute for Research on Women and Gender at the University of Michigan. Her work concerns the comparative investigation of race, sex, religion, and 'life', as these social categories manifest through the globalization of biomedical technologies. She has published on the social world of Ecuadorian *in-vitro* fertilization in *Culture Medicine and Psychiatry* (2006) and *American Ethnologist* (2007). Currently, she is revising this research for a monograph entitled *Equatorial* In-Vitro, *Reproductive Medicine and Modernity in Ecuador.* She is at the beginning of a new investigation on the transnational movements of intersex medicine.

Chloe Silverman is an Assistant Professor in the Science, Technology and Society Program at Penn State University, where she also teaches courses in Disability Studies. She is currently finishing a manuscript, *Autism, Love and Labor*, on the role of parent advocacy groups, and parental knowledge more generally, in research on autism spectrum disorders. The book examines the local, affect-laden practices that have worked to constitute autism as a diagnostic and clinical entity in a range of locations. Her cases include the Sonia Shankman Orthogenic School at the University of Chicago, the early years of the National

Society for Autistic Children, and contemporary groups such as the Autism Research Institute devoted to promoting biomedical interventions for autism.

Kaushik Sunder Rajan is Assistant Professor of Anthropology at the University of California, Irvine. His book, *Biocapital: The Constitution of Post-Genomic Life* (2006) is an ethnographic account of emergent drug development marketplaces in the United States and India in the context of new developments in genomics. He is currently researching the globalization of clinical trials, with a specific focus on the efforts to build clinical research infrastructure in India in anticipation of getting trials from Western biotech and pharmaceutical companies.

Acknowledgements

A great number of people have helped us to assemble this edited collection. In particular we would like to thank Nanneke Redclift, Sarah Franklin and Nikolas Rose for their institutional support and friendship in helping to bring this project together.

It has been a great pleasure to work with all authors who contributed to this book. Their enthusiasm, motivation and interest contributed significantly to giving this book its final form. Without doubt, this edited collection is a product of the conversations and discussions held at a workshop at the London School of Economics on 20 February 2006 titled 'Making Biosociality: Biologies and Identities in Formation'. We would like to express our appreciation to the Wellcome Trust's Biomedical Ethics Programme who provided us with generous funding to organize this event, which was as enjoyable as it was productive. The thoughtful comments and critical interventions of all the participants at this workshop gave us much pause for thought, greatly enhancing and enriching the form and content of this publication. We want to thank you all for taking the time to participate in this way.

Academic work does not take place in a vacuum – it is a product of the people you have around you. Carlos would like to express his gratitude to his colleagues at the London School of Economics and especially at the BIOS Centre for their friendship and encouragement over the years. He would especially like to thank Linsey McGoey, Ayo Wahlberg, Scott Vrecko, Chris Hamilton, David Reubi, Javier Lezaun and Filippa Lentzos. Patricia, Amaya and Isabel have provided the nourishing backdrop which makes the stuff of life so much the better. Sahra would like to thank friends and colleagues within and beyond the Anthropology Department at UCL for their on-going support and also acknowledge the ever-present encouragement of her family and partner.

Introduction

Biosocialities, genetics and the social sciences

Sahra Gibbon and Carlos Novas

The growth and expansion of certain fields of knowledge within the biological and medical sciences, including those linked to genomics, have widened the scope and range of techniques, theories and tools that can now be used to understand and intervene upon 'life'. Just as practitioners within these sciences have sought to develop new concepts and techniques by which to study and act upon vital biological processes, practitioners within the social sciences have also similarly engaged in the work of developing novel concepts and methods that are adequate to the task of analysing how potential transformations in understandings of 'life' may be involved in reassembling existing cultural, social, economic, ethical and political practices. This edited collection focuses on one idea developed in the early 1990s which has proved central to this task: Paul Rabinow's concept of *biosociality* (1992; 1996a)[1]. Critically interrogating this notion, the volume assesses its usefulness for examining a range of developments in the contemporary life sciences, whilst also thinking through how it may be put to work in new ways. The task here is not to offer a history of how the concept of *biosociality* emerged or how it has been taken up by sociologists and anthropologists, but rather to consider how it is theoretically and empirically valuable in the analysis of the biologies and socialities that are being assembled by a range of practitioners and social actors across a variety of interconnected sites such as laboratories, biotechnology companies, patients' organisations, medical clinics, biomedical charities and state institutions.

The widespread referencing of Rabinow's (1996a) concept of *biosociality* during the ten years since its original formulation illustrates its utility for many social scientists in mapping and investigating the transformations in knowledge and identity brought about by new genetic knowledge. Before outlining and summarising the thematic scope of this volume, we will begin by highlighting three conceptual arenas where the idea of biosociality has gained widespread currency; namely in reference to emergent identity practices, the re-framing of a distinction between nature/culture, and its heuristic approach to examining emergent and unfolding arenas of scientific inquiry. In discussing these three aspects we contextualise biosociality in relation to the concepts and theories which have pre-dated or co-evolved with this idea, in addition to the intellectual, social and scientific environment to which it responded and emerged from.

Perhaps the main reason why so many sociologists and anthropologists have been attracted to the concept of biosociality is that it has helped to think through how the emerging 'truths' that are being produced about humans in the diverse field of genetics shape our identities and forms of group activism. As Paul Rabinow (1996a) noted in his original essay, '… it is not hard to imagine groups formed around the chromosome 17, locus 16,256, site 654,376 allele variant with a guanine substitution. Such groups will have medical specialists, laboratories, narrative, traditions, and a heavy panoply of pastoral keepers to help them experience, share, intervene, and 'understand' their fate'. Whilst older forms of disease-related sociality and identity practices have existed in the past and continue to the present day, as a concept, biosociality was forged, as Rabinow notes in the afterword to this collection, to help think through what kinds of sociality could emerge at a time when understandings of what a disease is and the ways of acting upon illness were undergoing a process of considerable change.

Within the social sciences, much attention has been dedicated to mapping the extent to which the reclassification of many illnesses as being genetic in origin shapes individual and collective identity practices, exploring the implications of genetic knowledge for how individuals understand themselves or relate to others, and how persons affected by genetic conditions, through organizing themselves into groups, shape the production of knowledge about their conditions (Finkler, 2000; Gibbon, 2007; Konrad, 2005; Novas, 2006; Rabeharisoa and Callon, 2004; Rabinow, 1999; Rose and Novas, 2005; Taussig *et al.*, 2003). Biosociality has helped to speak to these diverse fields of inquiry. For instance, it helps to think about how the development of predictive genetic tests for conditions such as breast cancer or Huntington's disease alters experiences of illness, since these tests identify a susceptibility to a disease many years prior to the potential manifestation of symptoms. The status of being at genetic risk or the reclassification of a disease as being genetic in origin poses some profound questions in terms of how individuals identify themselves in relation to an illness and how they relate to similarly affected others. The creation of new opportunities for identifying with others who share a biological condition combined with the novel possibilities for acting upon disease has contributed to reshaping how patients organise themselves into groups and the kinds of activities that they undertake. At the same time, it is important to acknowledge that groups organised around genetic conditions existed in the past. These groups mostly concentrated on the provision of social and economic support to affected individuals and families, as well as the amelioration of clinical care given that there was little that could be done to treat these kinds of illnesses. However, the emergence of groups such as the Association Française contre les Myopathies (Rabeharisoa, 2003; Rabeharisoa and Callon, 2002; Rabeharisoa and Callon, 2004; Rabinow, 1999) and the Hereditary Disease Foundation, in the case of Huntington's disease (Wexler, 1996), provide illustrations of this shifting terrain. Over the course of the last three decades, such organisations have focused more on financing and directing scientific research efforts towards developing better understandings of their conditions, the creation of genetic tests, and ultimately, cures or therapies. These groups have not only managed to create new kinds of identities for patients, but more importantly, novel forms of bringing together patients, scientists, institutions, funds, and in some instances, biotechnology companies. Although it is a concept with antecedents in previous theoretical renderings of the relationship between identity and technology, such as Haraway's notion of the cyborg (1991), it could be said that the distinctiveness of *biosociality* lies in its attempts to name the kinds of socialities and identities that are forming around new sites of knowledge (genetics, molecular biology, genomics) and power (industrial, academic, medical).

The second key area where the concept of *biosociality* has had the most impact is in examining how transformations in the category of life contain the potential to dissolve the long established distinction between nature and culture. This is a theme that has been explored by others mainly in the field of STS with long standing interests in the modes of 'co-production' (Jasanoff, 2004) or networks (Callon, 1986) that create 'hybrid' (Latour, 1993) alignments between nature, science and society. The site which Rabinow concentrated on, in developing his ideas of *biosociality*, was the Human Genome Project – an international project to sequence all the genes in the human body. This project was in its infancy when this concept was coined in 1992, but it has now been completed and given rise to a number of successor projects such as proteomics, functional genomics, pharmacogenomics, and systems biology. For Rabinow the significance of this project lay in the fact that the object to be known – the human genome – would be known in such a way that it could be changed. He suggested this project was thoroughly modern: representing and intervening, knowledge and power, understanding and reform were built in from the start. What was significant about this project, from the perspective of the social sciences, was that the potential to know, remake and to create new life forms brought into question long established ideas of what counts as nature or natural. In this sense nature could no longer be considered as an entity or object which obeys its own laws and rhythms, but instead became a site that can be thoroughly assisted by human intervention, a place where reproduction could be technologically assisted and new forms of life could be created through the practice of science.

But as Paul Rabinow notes in his contribution (this volume), this concept was developed in order to stand in contrast to a then dominant term: socio-biology. Although socio-biology has come in many different forms and guises from the turn of the last century to the present, it consists of a range of knowledges and practices that are concerned with explaining the natural or biological determinants of human behaviour, culture and social order. At stake in socio-biology is an attempt to facilitate and engineer the construction of a more rational, efficient and scientifically ordered society based on understanding the evolutionary and biological forces that are claimed to have given rise to and which play a role in shaping human behaviour and sociality (Haraway, 1991). A key exemplar of this form of thinking is eugenics: eugenicists sought to create more rational, healthy and economically efficient societies through acting upon human reproduction. This is what Rabinow means when he claims that 'socio-biology … is a social project …' where 'the construction of society has been at stake' (Rabinow, 1996a).

By way of contrast, the concept of *biosociality* sought to work against forms of thought which posit a biological basis for society and culture. Such types of claims fail to take into account the diverse fields of knowledge (demography, statistics, social medicine, public health, sociology) and the range of practices (governmental, administrative, architectural, medical, militaristic, and industrial) through which the concept of society emerged over the course of the nineteenth century (Rabinow, 1989; Rose, 1996).

What is considered to be socially significant about advances in the field of molecular biology and the capacity to recombine DNA is that it serves to put into question what was once taken to be natural. Nature becomes a product of deliberate intervention: it becomes a locus of artificiality, an object produced by humans. In his essay, Rabinow (1996a) was concerned with thinking through how the new genetics contained the potential to put an end to the use of biology as a metaphor for modern society: alternatively, he proposed that the new genetics could become 'a circulation network of identity terms and restriction loci, around which and through which a new type of autoproduction will emerge which I call "biosociality"'. He then goes on to state:

> If sociobiology is culture constructed on the basis of a metaphor of nature, then in biosociality nature will be modelled on culture understood as practice. Nature will be known and remade through technique and will finally become artificial, just as culture becomes natural.
>
> (Rabinow, 1996a)

These statements suggest that if nature is understood as being artificial and culture is understood as a series of practices, then nature and culture are categories produced by human thought and actions. As such, with the advent of the new genetics, natural or bodily metaphors can no longer serve as an analogy for society, as they once prominently did in a range of sociological theories (for a good overview see: Levine, 1995). Alternatively, the new knowledges and techniques associated with the contemporary life sciences can constitute one axis or network, amongst many, through which individuals identify themselves, relate to others and engage in the artifice of modifying nature and the creation of social forms. This, we think, is what Rabinow means when he made the educated guess 'that the new genetics will prove to be a greater force for reshaping society and life than was the revolution in physics, because it will be embedded throughout the social fabric at the micro-level ...' (Rabinow, 1996a).

Paul Rabinow's (1996a) essay on *biosociality* is however of further interest and import due in part to its heuristic properties, reflecting an ethic of experimentation with theory and method in its concerns with describing and analysing the significance of developments in the life sciences across a number of social fields as they are in the process of emerging. This has been evident not only in Rabinow's analysis of the Human Genome Project, but is also present in his concern with studying the biotechnology industry as a key site to observe the development of novel understandings of life, new milieus or working conditions for scientists, and innovative modes for the infiltration of capitalism into the vital life processes of plants and organisms (Rabinow, 1996b). A large number of social scientists share a concern with examining how hype, hope and contingency are defining features of these novel 'assemblages' (Ong and Collier, 2005). That is examining the present(s) and near futures that are being created out of the merger of life and capital, science and technology, knowledge and power, how this contributes to reshaping how humans understand themselves or their relations to others, their experiences of health and illness and how local, national and global economies are being reorganised in this process (Cambrosio *et al.*, 2000; Franklin and Lock, 2003; Goodman *et al.*, 2003; Rose, 2001). Attention to the kinds of biologies and socialities that are unfolding and being unevenly and contingently assembled across a number of sites is an arena of inquiry shared by all the contributors to this volume. In taking these processes as the focus of their inquiry they draw on,whilst also extending, the heurism and ethic of experimentation in methodological and conceptual orientation that has been a defining feature of the concept of *biosociality.*

Six years after the completion of the first draft of the human genome, the rise of so called 'post-genomic' complexity, the eclipse of the status of 'the gene' (Lock, 2005), and the ever growing, yet still uneven global reach of genomics, we think that the time is right for reflection about the scope and limits of the notion of *biosociality.* In critically exemplifying, debating, historicising, re-situating and in some instances, refuting this concept, the collected essays in this volume make a timely contribution to broader collective efforts to theorise and empirically chart the relationships that figure between society and the life sciences. Through a combination of critical analysis, an engagement with old and new conceptual orientations within the fields of sociology and anthropology, and original empirical research conducted in a diverse range of social and national settings, this edited collection makes an intervention into thinking about the kinds of social, cultural and economic transformations that are at stake in relation to innovations in genomic knowledge and technology. The parameters for examining these issues are located at a dynamic interface between novel biological knowledges and technologies, social identities and forms of collective activism, the making and re-making of categories such as gender and race, the rise of biotechnological commerce, as well as transformations in long standing institutional cultures and states' practices relating to the provision of health care and the funding of science.

In critically engaging with and assessing the biosocial configurations of developments in a range of genomic and health biotechnologies we have identified four specific thematic arenas which we suggest cut across the collection of essays contained in this volume. These include (1) the intersection of novel identity practices with older modes of categorising persons based on class, gender or race; (2) the role of state and non-state actors or institutions including disease advocacy organisations and charities; (3) the production of 'novel' biomedical knowledges and technologies; and (4) the generation of wealth and commercial interests in biology and 'life itself'. Although conceptually delineated in the introduction to this volume all the chapters gathered here situate their analysis at the interface between two or more of these themes reflecting how a range of diverse, often seemingly contradictory arenas become newly significant and contingently assembled in the contemporary era of biological control. In this sense, the chapters in this book, like Rabinow's original conceptualisation of *biosociality,* illustrate how issues qualitatively different in scale and scope link the social and biological in a range of ways, becoming more or less temporarily or productively aligned.

Identity(ies) and identifications: the 'making up' of persons and personhood

The way that novel biological, genetic or medical knowledge and technologies shape identity and forms of identification has been a central topic of concern for some time in the social sciences where questions of agency, particularly in relation to female gender have been of long standing concern (Finkler, 2000; Franklin and Lock, 2003; Ginsburg and Rapp, 1995; Haraway, 1997; Lock and Kaufert, 1998; Rapp, 1999). It is significant that many of the contributors to this volume re-visit this issue in relation to what might be seen as an older medical technology, in-vitro fertilisation (IVF): a relatively well established medical intervention in many national settings, currently being given a novel gloss in relation to techniques such as prenatal genetic diagnosis (PGD), stem cell technologies, embryo and egg donation. In reflecting upon the concept of biosociality, many of the studies collated here therefore build on and honour the legacy of earlier work by examining how ideas of gender identity, the body, technology and science are caught up in mutually constituting and transforming ways.

In thinking through developments in the biological and genetic sciences, the authors contributing to this volume examine how in diverse arenas, older categories of classification based not only on gender, but also race or kinship inform, provide the framework for, or exist in tension with new kinds of biological identities. They powerfully illustrate Rabinow's (1996a) prescient point that older cultural categories have as much potential to be reinforced in relation to biosocial trajectories as novel modes of identity and identification (see also: Franklin *et al.,* 2000). For instance, we see here how particular entrenched ideas about female gender, relating to ideas of nurturance and care powerfully intersect with the quest for genetic knowledge and the pursuit of fundraising in a breast cancer research charity in the UK (Gibbon, this volume). Aditya Bharadwaj's chapter demonstrates how long standing cultural expectations and pressures to conceive for women in India are a defining and structuring feature of the way women's bodies are being made, in his terms, not biosocial but 'bio-available'. Elizabeth Roberts also contests the applicability of the notion of biosociality in her examination of the relation between female agency, identity and new biological interventions associated with the use of IVF in Ecuador. Here although ideas of modernity reflect the way that women are being constituted and constituting themselves as 'failed bodies', she argues that these modes of identification must also be understood in relation to deeply rooted historical, rather than contemporary, notions about the mutability of race.

For a number of other contributors recourse is made to Ian Hacking's (1992; 1995; 2002) notion of 'dynamic nominalism' as means of referencing how cultural categories linked to certain modes of identity making and biological knowledge become inter-relationally produced. As two chapters in this collection demonstrate, this notion seems particularly relevant in thinking about the 'making' up of persons in relation to the shifting terrains of scientific, genetic or medical knowledge and technology linked to autism and Alzheimer's disease (see chapters by Silverman and Lock respectively). Yet what is also powerfully reflected in many contributing chapters is the extent to which it is not only the productivity around identity making or modes of identification which is at stake in these developments, but also the 'unmaking' or dissolution of the person and/or the body. This is linked to the nature of the disease in the context of Alzheimer's disease (Lock, this volume), the structural inequalities that lead to the 'extraction' of persons and bodies in India (Bharadawaj, this volume) and the politics of pro-natalism in Israel where in one informant's felicitous phrasing the 'making of more disposable people' becomes an object and tool for ethnographic engagement (Nahman this volume). For some contributors the agentive modes of being biosocial are therefore less or not the only focus or object of import. Instead many highlight how the biological, in Agamben's (1998) terms the 'bare life' of persons, becomes quite literally diminished or resourced or sourced for different ends; a political economy of genomic knowledge and technology which many contributors see as an important dimension in understanding specific biosocial configurations. Some of these multi-layered complexities concerning agency and personhood are illustrated in Kaushik Sunder Rajan's discussion of the kind of 'experimental subjectivities' at stake in the recruitment of ex-mill workers near Bombay as trial subjects in the outsourcing of clinical trials to developing countries. His chapter brings a salutary reminder of the need for on-going monitoring of how forms of cultural classification and exploitation based on class and social location are binding to novel technologies and sciences.

Other contributors argue that the parameters of biosocial identity and identity making need to be expanded to describe and reflect the practices under examination. Attending more specifically to questions of 'patienthood' in an era of developments in genomic knowledge and technology, some chapters point to how it is less the sick individual who is the active identifying or identifiable agent in particular social arenas, but rather what have been described as 'proxy' patients or patient representatives (Landzelius and Dumit, 2006). This is illustrated in both Sahra Gibbon's discussion of the way the BRCA carrier becomes an *iconic* figure in the context of breast cancer activism and Chloe Silverman's analysis of how a discourse of heredity in relation to autism leads to parents '(re)discovering' their own autistic tendencies following their child's diagnosis. In highlighting these expanded networks of biosocial involvement there is also an interesting intersecting trajectory between an examination of the way that notions of 'affect', 'care' and 'memorialisation' recruit not just the sick individual but also family, friends and non-related others into differently productive alignments. Collectively these chapters point to a need for examining the distributed parameters of various more or less biosocial networks that encompass not just the figure of the 'patient', raising questions about the boundaries of patienthood in an era of biosocial identity making.

Institutional parameters: the state and non-state actors

Focusing less on the individualising scope (or the limits) of identificatory modes associated with biosociality, others have turned to the collectivising potential and institutional contexts through which developments in the life sciences are unfolding. Perhaps one of the most emblematic areas where this has been explored is in relation to the growth of a range of disease advocacy organisations (Callon and Rabeharisoa, 2003; Epstein, 2007; Novas, 2006; Rabeharisoa, 2003; Rabeharisoa and Callon, 2002, 2004). Some of these groups are not only now demanding a say in biomedical research, but are increasingly also contributing towards its funding and coordination, generating what has been described as 'research in the wild' (Rabeharisoa 2003). Yet the social forms by which patients' or advocates' experiences, knowledge or hopes become linked to laboratory research in comparative international arenas are themselves varied with differing consequences for institutional structures and practices.

Novel forms of what might be described as 'lay expertise', 'activism' and/or 'citizenship' are discernible in some of the case studies examined here where there are identifiable transformations in the types of institutional relations that prevail between patients, medical professionals and scientists. Building on work in the social sciences which has examined a lay/scientific interface in relation to emergent health technologies (Lock *et al.*, 2000; Rapp, 1999) these studies raise questions about an assumed and/or static binary divide between patients and practitioners. The chapters by Chloe Silverman and Carlos Novas provide empirical illustrations of how a variety of different patient advocates in the fields of autism and rare health conditions such as Pompe disease, have been and continue to be involved in directing, resourcing, and the funding of genetic research, as well as the way that health professionals and scientists are caught up in these developments.

Yet it is salutary to be reminded that although the numbers of such patient groups have expanded in the last twenty years, in certain disease domains, they are not necessarily novel or uniformly similar (Hess, 2004a, 2004b). Alliances between specific publics and scientists have characterised differing moments of the twentieth century in Europe and America, with 'wars' against tuberculosis, polio and cancer enabling and mobilising these endeavours with varying success (see Austoker, 1989; Löwy, 1996 in relation to cancer). Heeding the need for a more historicised perspective a number of the chapters in this collection bring a temporal dimension to their examination of disease advocacy. They show how and the variable extent to which the new genetics has configured the context and content of existing patients' organisations, recognising that many of these groups existed prior to the revolution in contemporary biotechnology (see chapters by Lock, Gibbon, Silverman, Novas, this volume). An important insight generated by the bringing together of these various forms of patient activism is therefore to demonstrate the huge diversity of responses to recent developments in genetics and in relation to the impact this has had for different disease advocacy groups. As Margaret Lock points out (this volume) the biological history and social character of any particular disease and its biomedical classification has consequences for the kinds of biosocial configurations that coalesce around recent genetic discoveries.

The comparative international arenas examined in this volume also bring to bear an important perspective on how innovations in the biomedical sciences intersect with state actors and institutions. This includes state or national policies concerning health and identity. It is an interface which is powerfully illustrated in Michal Nahman's timely examination of pro-natalist policies in relation to the provision of IVF and egg donation in the context of the 'Intifada' on the West Bank. Her description of different 'bio-social' moments become a resource in demonstrating the 'synecdochic ricochets' that link the micro-practices of extraction, fertilisation and implantation in the IVF clinic to Israeli state practices of 'transfer', 'citizenship' and 'naturalisation'. The role of the state also looms large in Bharadwaj's examination of the use of IVF and stem cell technologies in India where the rise of 'Neo-India' is an important instrumental backdrop to examining how the pursuit of 'modernising' technologies continue to sustain what he sees as entrenched inequalities and deprivations, despite the widening of access to such 'modern' interventions'. If it is the instrumentalising role of state actors which is a focus of concern for some, for others, it is the absence of health or welfare provision (Roberts, this volume) or the way organisations more normally positioned outside of or in opposition to the 'state', such as charity (Gibbon), which come to define the meeting point between the biological and social under examination. Here we see the varying ways that state and non-state actors respond, enable, legitimise and inform the garnering of resources, and help or hinder the translation of novel biomedical techniques into clinical practice.

The production of 'novel' biological knowledge and technologies

A third cross-cutting theme explored in this edited collection, as part of an examination of biosociality, is how and to what extent advances in the life sciences are bringing into being novel technologies, materialities and objects for the production of truth about vital life processes. This is a process that Paul Rabinow (1996a) provocatively highlighted in his own work where he indicated that alongside the Human Genome Project there 'are adjacent enterprises and institutions in which and through which new understandings, new practices, and new technologies of labour and life will certainly be articulated: prime among them the biotechnology industry.' All of the contributors to this volume share a concern for examining the material conditions and processes through which scientific knowledge, biomedical technologies and novel life forms are produced in a diverse array of cultural, institutional and national settings. At the same time there is recognition that the biological is and has always been a 'locally' produced category with comparative historical and cultural guises (Lock, 1993; Lock and Kaufert, 2001). This is brought to the fore particularly in relation to Elizabeth Roberts' work in Ecuador where she points out how the historical embeddedness of ideas around a mutable biology have been central to conceptions of 'race' in this national context, informing and influencing the meaning and uptake of reproductive interventions such as IVF.

It is important to acknowledge that one of the principal reasons why recent developments in the life sciences have provided a fertile ground for social scientific inquiry is because they appear to put into question many taken-for-granted assumptions about the nature of science. Whilst in the past it was possible for social scientists to maintain clear cut distinctions between 'pure' and 'applied' science, these type distinctions have fortuitously started to fade into obsolescence. The ascendance of fields such as molecular biology has led to the blurring of these distinctions. As Kaushik Sunder Rajan (this volume) notes in his discussion of biosociality and pharmacogenomics in India, reconfigurations in the epistemologies of how life is understood and known are implicated in new forms of labour and capitalist accumulation strategies. He productively discusses how capital and intensive funding is a fundamental condition of possibility for the contemporary conduct of academic or private life science research. Of course, the specific modalities and forms that capital takes, the specific character which life science research assumes, and the processes through which 'experimental' subjects are constituted are profoundly shaped by local ecologies and histories within which it operates.

A number of chapters contained in this edited collection focus more specifically on examining how lay persons and genetic advocacy groups can help bring into being new sorts of materialities, technologies and scientific practices, which in turn, serve to further fuel collective action. This can include the raising of funds for scientific research, the design of scientific studies, the management of collaborations between laboratories, but also in some instances, the establishment of collections of blood, tissue and DNA. As Chloe Silverman's (this volume) detailed research exquisitely shows, parents of autistic children have invested significantly in the hope and promise associated with the contemporary life sciences. They have created organisations dedicated to financing scientific research efforts and to creating a resource essential to the production of knowledge about the biological basis of autism – a blood and tissue bank known as the Autism Genetic Resource Exchange. This blood and tissue bank is not only a resource that may one day lead to the elucidation of the genetic basis of autism, but it also serves as an important locale to bring together persons affected by this condition, and an important resource that Cure Autism Now is able to use to influence the direction of scientific research and the distribution of any economic or therapeutic benefits derived from it. The benefits derived from research on conditions such as autism may extend well beyond this particular illness. This theme is developed in Carlos Novas' chapter where he discusses how research by a biotechnology company, set up by the father of two children affected by a rare condition known as Pompe disease, had the potential to be applied to a total of forty-eight other disorders which share a similar biological pathway. A number of social scientists have noted (Rapp, 2003; Rapp *et al.*, 2002) how genes and their associated biological pathways can serve as one route for the creation of alliances between disease advocacy organisations. As we will discuss more extensively in the following section, these biological pathways can serve as a significant source for the generation of wealth.

Yet whilst it is often tempting to think of and describe developments in the life sciences in terms of epochs, revolutions or epistemological breaks, it is also useful to think of these developments in terms of a process of succession and gradual change. Moreover, while advances in the life sciences have in some respects put into question established forms of thought and ways of doing science or medicine, as the concept of biosociality attests, the old and the new can co-exist and co-mingle with one another in highly interesting ways. For instance, Margaret Lock's chapter urges caution in thinking about the impact that the new genetics has had on understanding the disease aetiology of Alzheimer's. Whilst the biological and molecular pathways which underlie this disease are no doubt being profoundly investigated, more established forms of thinking about Alzheimer's disease are still very prominent and significant for the families and carers of persons affected by this condition. These types of concerns are also very evident in Chloe Silverman's chapter where some parents and patients' groups actively contribute to the development of knowledge about autism and ways of acting upon this condition that are not rooted in the contemporary life sciences. These forms of knowledge are no less legitimate or less advanced than that which goes on in molecular biology laboratories: their research object is simply different and does not register as prominently on social, political and economic agendas.

In fact the changing medical aetiologies of the different diseases examined in this collection bring a range of scientific objects into and out of focus, such that the ideas and materialities of brains, genes and social environment inter-digitate with temporal shifts in the forms of health activism around these conditions. In the case of autism these shifts in biological aetiology serve to constitute the condition as a 'spectrum' disorder; a classification which as Silverman points out 'loops' back to help identify and mobilise the identificatory practices of various 'activist' populations. By way of contrast, shifts in the 'genetic' aetiology and ability to predict the onset of Alzheimer's have, as Margaret Lock points out, 'blocked' biosociality based on a sense of 'shared DNA', at least in part due to the increasingly recognised complexity of the disease aetiology and gene-environment pathways which has the effect of rendering predictive knowledge neither possible or useful. It is interesting to note that a different but equally complex, yet somewhat hype filled arena of breast cancer genetics has been more readily and swiftly translated out of research arenas and into the clinical domain (Gibbon, 2007). This suggests that the biosocialities of being (or more usually the risk of being) a BRCA carrier meld not only with diverse domains of activism in relation to breast cancer but align techniques, research objects and bodily matter in ways that are differently configured in relation to conditions such as Alzheimer's disease; a differentiation that must be recognised and explored further in relation to a variety of disease conditions.

The generation of wealth through biology

The final cross cutting theme explored in this edited collection is the relationship between the life sciences and the economy. From the early 1970s onwards, it could be said that life became economically valuable in entirely new ways through the combination of the development of novel scientific techniques which enabled DNA to be moved from one species to another and the emergence of a significant industry organised around biotechnology. Within the social sciences, the commercialisation of scientific research, the development of property rights in life itself, and the dynamics of the biotechnology industry have constituted topics of considerable concern (Andrews and Nelkin, 2001; Gold, 1996; Hayden, 2003; Parry, 2004; Rabinow, 1996b, 1999; Rose, 2006; Sunder Rajan, 2006; Thackray, 1998; Yoxen, 1983). Although it would be all too easy to assume that the relationship between the life sciences and the economy is unidirectional, as the content of many of the chapters in this collection richly document, economic conditions, market opportunities, state policies and ethical regimes shape the practice and content of basic scientific research. The accounts produced in these chapters suggest that the types of relationships that transpire between science, medicine and the market are dynamic, fluid and global in scope. This field is also fraught with tension, ambiguity and uncertainty: the potential of the life sciences to assist human reproduction or augment health often challenges or runs up against existing cultural values and practices. A theme that runs throughout many of the chapters brought together under the rubric of this collection is how what is at stake in the development of the biotechnology industry and the promotion of the life sciences is the construction of particular kinds of economies and societies.

One of the most vexing and interesting challenges presented to social scientists studying the life sciences has been to develop conceptual tools adequate to considering the forms through which life itself has become economically valuable and the implications that this has for how we consider the body and its constituent parts. Building upon concepts such as biovalue (Waldby, 2000, 2002) and ethical biocapital (Franklin, 2003; Franklin and Lock, 2003) a number of chapters in this volume reflect on how vital life processes and parts of human bodies are being remade and harnessed in order to generate viable business strategies, novel products and profits. Whilst human body parts have been generative of value in the past in terms of their capacity to augment human health and generate wealth through their transformation into knowledge or information (Lock, 2001; Waldby, 2000, 2002), the techniques associated with the contemporary life sciences enable blood, tissue and DNA to become economically valuable and useful for the enhancement of human vitality in entirely new ways. As Aditya Bharadwaj captures in his essay, bodies are open to new practices of 'extraction and insertion'. With the advent of reproductive and genetic technologies, entities such as embryos, stem cells, or DNA become available for use and circulation in medical, gift and market economies. As in all economies, the social practices through which body parts are alienated are globally uneven and inequitable – the conditions and compensation received in relation to these extractive processes are significantly different in Indian slums than in American suburbs. Of course, the counterpoint of extraction, is insertion, as Bhardawaj notes. Today, the body is increasingly being constructed as open to repair and intervention through an entirely new range of technologies which seek to work on the body at the molecular and genetic level. A pressing issue for sociological and anthropological analysis is whose bodies are open to genetic and molecular remedies. In India, there is great disparity over the social position of those whose bodies' embryos, cells and tissues are extracted, in contrast to the persons into whom they are inserted. As Carlos Novas comments in his contribution, enzyme replacement therapies are predominately inserted into the bodies of children who live in Australasia, North America and Japan, contributing even further to global health inequities.

Another reason why so many social scientists have been drawn to analyse the intersection between science and markets is that it poses some profound questions about the contemporary conditions for the production of knowledge and truth. Today, the production of truth in the life sciences is increasingly dependent upon the generation of intellectual property rights, intensive funding, state support, and capital – a topic that is richly discussed by Kaushik Sunder Rajan in his chapter. As we attempted to outline in the previous section, the production of biomedical knowledge does not exclusively take place in universities, but increasingly in biotechnology companies, the social forms and networks created by lay persons and disease advocacy organisations, or, in some instances, a combination of all of the above. This is evidenced in Carlos Novas' contribution to this volume where he explores how a father with two children affected by Pompe disease not only established a disease advocacy organisation, but also helped to found a biotechnology firm dedicated to finding a cure for his children's illness. Although this example is highly unusual, it serves to illustrate how non-scientists can actively contribute to one of the prominent organisational forms through which biomedical knowledge and therapies are produced. At the present moment, the large amounts of capital that are required to bring new biological therapies into being can only be successfully mobilised by biotechnology firms and pharmaceutical companies. And of course, the ability to successfully mobilise capital is dependent on the capacity to turn vital life processes into a resource for the production of wealth.

As the biotechnology industry has grown in scale and economic significance, so too has the interest of social scientists in mapping the dynamics and contours of this industry as it unfolds. Sociologists and anthropologists have dedicated considerable attention to analysing the scientific, technical, legal, social, economic and political circumstances which have contributed to the assemblage of this industry on a national and global scale. Of course, the configuration and assemblage of this industry has shown considerable national variation and has unfolded at different historical paces as Sunder Rajan explains in his contribution to this volume. Within the context of India, the development of the pharmaceutical and biotechnology industry is being shaped by the recent entry of this country into the WTO, but is also being heavily invested in by capital that was previously oriented around the textile trade. Aditya Bhardawaj's description of Neo-India is particularly apt at capturing how the promotion of the biotechnology industry forms an important component of contemporary state strategies to rejuvenate their economies through the mobilisation of the reproductive capacities of living organisms.

A significant rationale which informs the novel alliances that are being forged between the life sciences and the market is the potential for biotechnology to develop new means of acting upon the health of the citizenry. The merger between health and industry, central to governmental rationalities throughout the nineteenth and twentieth centuries, is being contemporaneously reconfigured. This development is brought out in Carlos Novas' chapter which focuses on the creation of substantial political economies oriented around extremely rare diseases. The creation and existence of these political economies demonstrates how firms and the markets can, with the aid of legislation, be used to correct one of its inequities, that is, its previous failure to develop treatments for rare conditions. As further evidenced by Elizabeth Roberts and Aditya Bhardawaj's chapters, there is strong consumer interest and demand in the hope and promise of contemporary genetics to assist human reproduction or develop novel methods for diagnosing and treating illness. As Novas discusses, these hopes are increasingly being shaped by the ever more sophisticated marketing tactics of pharmaceutical and biotechnology companies. These and other chapters in the collection point to a complex interpenetration between biosociality, commerce, institutional arrangements, forms of identity making, and biopolitics.

Conclusion

In empirically outlining how, where and in what ways the concept of biosociality does and does not provide a useful means of thinking through or even describing the kinds of relationships that exist between the biological and the social, the chapters brought together under the rubric of this volume bring to the fore a diverse, diffuse and rich set of social and cultural practices. Although Rabinow's much referenced concept of *biosociality* has provided a reflective starting point for this collection, the chapters collated here bring a much needed diversity to an understanding of the way that different *biosocialities* are brought to bear in a range of comparative arenas. Here the question of novelty, as well as ideas of contingency, are not only subject to renewed critical scrutiny but are themselves brought into productive interface with what Sunder Rajan (this volume) usefully terms the multiple 'over-determinations' associated with these developments. Indeed an important feature of this book is the way that a number of its contributors shed light on the spaces, practices and persons which they suggest a notion of biosociality has 'failed to account for' (Bharadwaj, this volume). For others, the multi-layered complexity and inherent ambiguity of the notion of biosociality has and continues to provide a useful entry point for examining these developments, which invites and encourages innovation in method, concept and critical analysis.

From this perspective, Rabinow's (1996a) original conceptual orientation is by turns or sometimes simultaneously, a descriptive tool for both current and prospective developments and/or a contested empirical and conceptual orientation that exists in tension with different ways of configuring the biological and social in comparative historical and cultural arenas. The collection does not only represent a varied and richly detailed empirical intervention in understanding developments in the field of genomics, but brings new concepts, methods and theories to bear, while also recognising the on-going import and salience of older cultural categories and theoretical orientations. Here discussions of 'bio-availability' or 'bio-crossing', 'experimental subjectivity' or 'synechdochic ricochets', to name a few of the novel conceptual re-workings developed by contributors to this collection, sit in productive tension with discussion of the role of the state and inequities linked to gender, race and class. In this sense the range of interpretative approaches represented by the eight essays contained in this collection is not only a testament to the richly varied theoretical and empirical content of the individual chapters but also reflects the original experimental orientation engendered by the concept of biosociality. One of the most significant and perhaps lasting legacies of Rabinow's idea is the concept of *biosociality* as an orientation that invites innovation in method and theory in thinking about the way the social and biological are being (co)-configured in relation to developments in the life sciences. It is a spirit of experimentation which the book honours and will we hope in turn inform and provide further fuel for those grappling with the biosocialities of evolving fields of genomic knowledge and technology.

Note

1 Paul Rabinow's essay titled 'Artificiality and enlightenment: from sociobiology to biosociality' originally appeared in J. Crary and S. Kwinter (1992), *Zone 6: Incorporations*, New York: Zone. As this book is not available in all libraries, we make reference throughout the edited collection to a latter version of this essay which appeared in P. Rabinow (1996), *Essays on the Anthropology of Reason*, Princeton, NJ: Princeton University Press.

References

Agamben, G. (1998) *Homo Sacer: Sovereign Power and Bare Life*, Stanford, CA: Stanford University Press.

Andrews, L. and Nelkin, D. (2001) *Body Bazaar: The Market for Human Tissue in Biotechnology Age*, New York: Crown Publishers.

Austoker, J. (1989) *A History of the Imperial Cancer Research Fund 1902–1986*, Oxford: Oxford University Press.

Callon, M. (1986) 'Some elements of a sociology of translation: domenstication of the scallops and fisherman of St. Brieuc's Bay' in J.Law (ed.) *Power, Action and Belief: A New Sociology of Knowledge? Sociological Review* Monograph No 32 Keele: University of Keele Press.

Callon, M. and Rabeharisoa, V. (2003) 'Gino's lesson on humanity: genetics, mutual entanglements and the sociologist's role', *Economy and Society*, 33, 1: 1–27.

Cambrosio, A., Lock, M. and Young, A. (eds) (2000) *Living and Working with the New Medical Technologies: Intersections of Inquiry*, Cambridge: Cambridge University Press.

Epstein, S. (2007) 'Patient groups and health movements', in Hackett, E.J., Amsterdamska, O., Lynch, M. and Wajcman, J. (eds) *New Handbook of Science and Technology Studies*, Cambridge, MA: MIT Press.

Finkler, K. (2000) *Experiencing the New Genetics: Family and Kinship on the Medical Frontier*, Philadelphia, PA: University of Pennsylvania Press.

Franklin, S. (2003) 'Ethical biocapital: new strategies of cell culture', in Franklin, S. and Lock, M. (eds) *Remaking Life and Death: Toward an Anthropology of the Biosciences*, Oxford: James Currey.

Franklin, S., Lury, C. and Stacey, J. (2000) *Global Nature, Global Culture*, London: Sage.

Franklin, S. and Lock, M.M. (eds) (2003) *Remaking Life and Death: Toward an Anthropology of the Biosciences*, Oxford: James Currey.

Gibbon, S. (2007) *Breast Cancer Genes and the Gendering of Knowledge*, London: Palgrave Macmillan.

Ginsburg, F.D. and Rapp, R. (eds) (1995) *Conceiving the New World Order: The Global Politics of Reproduction*, Berkeley, CA: University of California Press.

Gold, E.R. (1996) *Body Parts: Property Rights and the Ownership of Human Biological Materials*, Washington, DC: Georgetown University Press.

Goodman, A.H., Heath, D. and Lindee, M.S. (eds) (2003) *Genetic Nature/Culture: Anthropology and Science beyond the Two-Culture Divide*, Berkeley, CA: University of California Press.

Hacking, I. (1992) 'World-making by kind-making: child abuse for example', in Douglas, M. and Hull, D. (eds) *How Classification Works: Nelson Goodman among the Social Sciences*, Edinburgh: Edinburgh University Press.

Hacking, I. (1995) 'The looping effects of human kinds', in Sperber, D., Premack, D. and Premack, A.J. (eds) *Causal Cognition: A Multi-Disciplinary Approach*, Oxford: Clarendon Press.

Hacking, I. (2002) *Historical Ontology*, Cambridge, MA: Harvard University Press.

Haraway, D. (1991) *Simians, Cyborgs, and Women: The Reinvention of Nature*, New York: Routledge.

Haraway, D.J. (1997) *Modest-Witness@Second-Millennium. FemaleMan-meets-OncoMouse: Feminism and Technoscience*, New York: Routledge.

Hayden, C.P. (2003) *When Nature Goes Public: The Making and Unmaking of Bioprospecting in Mexico*, Princeton, NJ: Princeton University Press.

Hess, D.J. (2004a) 'Health, the environment and social movements', *Science as Culture*, 13, 4: 421–7.

Hess, D.J. (2004b) 'Medical modernisation, scientific research fields and the epistemic politics of health social movements', *Sociology of Health and Illness*, 26, 6: 695–709.

Jasanoff, S. (2004) *States of Knowledge; The Co-Production of Science and the Social Order*, London: Routledge

Konrad, M. (2005) *Narrating the New Predictive Genetics: Ethics, Ethnography and Science*, Cambridge: Cambridge University Press.

Landzelius, K. and Dumit, J. (2006) 'Introduction: patient organization movements and new metamorphoses in patienthood', *Social Science and Medicine*, 62, 3: 529–37.

Latour, B.(1993) *We Have Never Been Modern* (trans by C. Porter), London: Harvester Wheatsheaf

Levine, D.N. (1995) 'The organism metaphor in sociology', *Social Research*, 62, 2: 239–65.

Lock, M. (1993) *Encounters with Aging: Mythologies of Menopause in Japan and North America*, Berkeley, CA: University of California Press.

Lock, M. (2001) 'The alienation of body tissue and the biopolitics of immortalized cell lines', *Body and Society*, 7, 2–3: 63–91.

Lock, M. (2005) 'Eclipse of the gene and the return of divination', *Current Anthropology*, 46: Supplement, S47–S70.

Lock, M. and Kaufert, P.A. (2001) 'Menopause, local biologies, and cultures of aging', *American Journal of Human Biology*, 13, 4: 494–504.

Lock, M. and Kaufert, P.A. (eds) (1998) *Pragmatic Women and Body Politics*, New York: Cambridge University Press.

Lock, M., Young, A. and Cambrosio, A. (eds) (2000) *Living and Working with the New Medical Technologies: Intersections of Inquiry*, Cambridge: Cambridge University Press.

Löwy, I. (1996) *Between Bench and Bedside: Science, Healing, and Interleukin-2 in a Cancer Ward*, Cambridge, MA: Harvard University Press.

Novas, C. (2006) 'The political economy of hope: patients' organizations, science and biovalue', *BioSocieties*, 1, 3: 289–305.

Ong, A. and Collier, S.J. *Global Assemblages: Technology, Politics, and Ethics as Anthropological Problems,* Malden, MA: Blackwell.

Parry, B. (2004) *Trading the Genome: Investigating the Commodification of Bio-information*, New York: Columbia University Press.

Rabeharisoa, V. (2003) 'The struggle against neuromuscular diseases in France and the emergence of the "partnership model" of patient organisation', *Social Science and Medicine*, 57, 11: 2127–36.

Rabeharisoa, V. and Callon, M. (2002) 'The involvement of patients' associations in research', *International Social Science Journal*, 171: 57–65.

Rabeharisoa, V. and Callon, M. (2004) 'Patients and scientists in French muscular dystrophy research', in Jasanoff, S. (ed.) *States of Knowledge: The Co-production of Science and Social Order*, London: Routledge.

Rabinow, P. (1989) *French Modern: Norms and Forms of the Social Environment*, Cambridge, MA: MIT Press.

Rabinow, P. (1992) 'Artificiality and enlightenment: from sociobiology to biosociality', in Crary, J. and Kwinter, S. (eds) *Zone 6: Incorporations*, New York: Zone.

Rabinow, P. (1996a) 'Artificiality and enlightenment: from sociobiology to biosociality', *Essays on the Anthropology of Reason*, Princeton, NJ: Princeton University Press.

Rabinow, P. (1996b) *Making PCR: A Story of Biotechnology*, Chicago, IL: University of Chicago Press.

Rabinow, P. (1999) *French DNA: Trouble in Purgatory*, Chicago, IL: University of Chicago Press.

Rapp, R. (1999) *Testing Women, Testing the Fetus: The Social Impact of Amniocentesis in America*, New York: Routledge.

Rapp, R. (2003) 'Cell life and death, child life and death: genomic horizons, genetic diseases, family stories', in Franklin, S. and Lock, M.M. (eds) *Remaking Life and Death: Toward an Anthropology of the Biosciences*, Oxford: James Currey.

Rapp, R., Taussig, K.S. and Heath, D. (2002) 'Genealogical disease: where hereditary abnormality, biomedical explanation, and family responsibility meet', in Franklin, S.

and McKinnon, S. (eds) *Relative Matters: New Directions in Kinship Study*, Durham, NC: Duke University Press.

Rose, N. (1996) 'The death of the social? Re-figuring the territory of government', *Economy and Society*, 25, 3: 327–56.

Rose, N. (2001) 'The politics of life itself', *Theory, Culture and Society*, 18, 6: 1–30.

Rose, N. (2006) *The Politics of Life Itself: Biomedicine, Power, and Subjectivity in the Twenty-First Century*, Princeton, NJ: Princeton University Press.

Rose, N. and Novas, C. (2005) 'Biological citizenship', in Ong, A. and Collier, S. (eds) *Global Assemblages: Technology, Politics, and Ethics as Anthropological Problems*, Malden, MA: Blackwell.

Sunder Rajan, K. (2006) *Biocapital: The Constitution of Postgenomic Life*, Durham, NC: Duke University Press.

Taussig, K.S., Rapp, R. and Heath, D. (2003) 'Flexible eugenics: technologies of the self in the age of genetics', in Goodman, A.H., Heath, D. and Lindee, M.S. (eds) *Genetic Nature/Culture: Anthropology and Science beyond the two-culture divide*, Berkeley CA: University of California Press.

Thackray, A. (1998) *Private Science: Biotechnology and the rise of the Molecular Sciences*, Philadelphia, PA: University of Pennsylvania Press.

Waldby, C. (2000) *The Visible Human Project: Informatic Bodies and Posthuman Medicine*, London and New York: Routledge.

Waldby, C. (2002) 'Stem cells, tissue cultures and the production of biovalue', *Health: An Interdisciplinary Journal for the Social Study of Health, Illness and Medicine*, 6, 3: 305–23.

Wexler, A. (1996) *Mapping Fate: A Memoir of Family, Risk and Genetic Research*, Berkeley, CA: University of California Press.

Yoxen, E. (1983) *The Gene Business: Who Should Control Biotechnology*, New York: Harper and Row.

1 Charity, breast cancer activism and the iconic figure of the BRCA carrier

Sahra Gibbon

Introduction

The burgeoning growth in health activism around breast cancer since the early 1990s has been facilitated by and led to a proliferation of patient, lay or grass roots breast cancer organisations in both the UK, Europe and North America. All have in different ways contributed to the de-stigmatisation of the disease by highlighting the scale of the breast cancer 'epidemic', informing a discourse about 'risk' and the need for 'awareness' (Anglin 1997; Montini 1996; Lantz and Booth 1998; Klawiter 2000; Potts 1999; Blackstone 2004; King 2001). Glossed collectively in terms of 'breast cancer activism' the diverse social collectives that come together under the rubric of this descriptive term are illustrative of the way, as Epstein points out, the 'politics of feminist and women's health criss-cross the bio-medical landscape' such that they are now 'implicated with rise of pat groups and health movements to quite an astonishing degree' (2007: 8).

This is in part why the cultural arenas which constitute the 'breast cancer movement' provide an important social space in which to examine the forms of biosociality linked to the identification of two inherited susceptibility genes associated with breast cancer in the mid-1990s. In pre-dating these genomic 'discoveries' *and* evolving not only in relation to but to a large extent also outside developments in genetic knowledge and technology, the social and cultural practices linked to breast cancer activism provide a context in which to critically explore the particular scope and shape of biosociality at stake in these developments. By addressing this interface the chapter builds on the work of others who have pointed to the productive link between the growing culture of health activism in relation to breast cancer and the translation from the lab to the clinic of the knowledges and technologies associated with two inherited susceptibility genes, BRCA 1 and 2 in the mid- and late 1990s (Parathasarthy 2003; Kaufert 2003; Cartwright 2000; see also Gibbon 2007). This discussion, examining the shifting temporalities of genetic knowledge and health activism around breast cancer, sheds fresh light on this interface by outlining what kind of intervention the discoveries and application of the knowledge and technologies associated with the 'BRCA genes' constitute for a particular nexus of individuals within the breast cancer 'movement' in the UK. Focusing on the social relations and cultural practices in a breast cancer research charity it examines how diffuse or distributed yet powerful gendered articulations of bio-sociality and citizenship are brought about at the junction between genes, technologies and persons.

Locating bio-sociality outside the clinic

The identification of two inherited susceptibility genes in the mid-1990s, BRCA1/2, associated with an increased risk of developing breast cancer not only received an inordinate amount of media and public attention (Henderson and Kitzinger 1999) but has also in many ways been something of a cornerstone and a test case in an emerging field of predictive medicine. The 'overwhelming' number of referrals in the mid- to late 1990s to regional genetic clinics in the UK, for those considered to be at risk of breast cancer, has been one if not *the* determining factor in the setting up of specialist and dedicated cancer genetic clinics and the institutionalisation of a triage system to manage the large numbers of those seeking or being referred (Wonderling *et al.* 2001). Given what might be seen as this 'demand', there is an assumption that large numbers of women are being identified as carriers of the two BRCA genes and that this is a situation that warrants at the same time that it makes evident the importance of investigating the bio-social identities that gene 'carrier' status might be thought to bring about.

The way developments in genetic knowledge have implications for the identities of those so-called 'patients' and their families caught up in predictive health care, have been explored elsewhere, both in relation to breast cancer (Hallowell 1999; d'Agin-Court Canning 2001; Gibbon 2007) as well as other conditions where genes are thought to be involved (Konrad 2005; Rapp 1999). The bio-socialities associated with the discovery and application of knowledge linked to the BRCA genes, that are the focus of this chapter, are somewhat differently positioned. Not withstanding the importance of research exploring the experiences over the long term of the currently relatively small numbers of persons who are or have relatives who are positively identified as carriers of the gene, I would argue that to limit research to the bio-socialities of this small, and for the moment, somewhat exceptional group distorts and misapprehends how BRCA genetics has emerged at the forefront of predictive medicine in the UK.[1] For these reasons I would suggest that the conjunction between the biological and social brought about by and which have helped propel developments in BRCA genetics must be located in broader social arenas.

Given the potential scope and reach of developments in genetic knowledge *and* the burgeoning growth of the breast cancer movement over the last 10 years, it is perhaps not surprising that the interface between BRCA genetics and breast cancer activism plays out not just at the clinical interface but also outside this medical domain.[2] This chapter explores the synergies and tensions between sciences and publics generated by these developments through examining the interface between a specific sort of patient or lay activism and the pursuit of genetic research in one institutional arena within the broad and diverse spectrum of groups and communities that are part of the so-called breast cancer movement in the UK. Drawing on ethnographic research with a high profile breast cancer research charity, this chapter plots how the field of research characterised in terms of 'the genetics of breast cancer' has a powerful productive presence while also itself being instrumentalised at the interface between breast cancer 'activism' and charitably funded breast cancer research. It shows how the gendered risk, hope and need represented by the *iconic* figure of the female BRCA carrier is central to this task, implicated in and instrumental to the 'making up' of a certain kind of breast cancer activist. In examining therefore how the biosocialities of BRCA genetics operate in a broader terrain of breast cancer the chapter underlines the need to engage with disjuncture in the shifting terrain of genomic and post-genomic interventions, novelty and stasis in the different *gendered* modes of identity making and identification caught up with these developments and the way long standing institutional cultures, such as charity in the UK, provide a structuring context for particular bio-social configurations.

In elucidating these shifts the chapter plots a very deliberate temporal trajectory that draws on ethnographic research with a breast cancer charity from 1999 to 2001, as well as more recent research. Three key ethnographic excerpts become the starting point for discussion of the shifting bio-socialities of BRCA genetics, exemplifying in each case how the *iconic* figure of the BRCA carrier is more or less productively situated.

Memorialisation and genetics as redemptory knowledge

It is early morning in west London in April 1999. I am standing inside the charity's newly opened research centre waiting for the start of what are known as the 'monthly tours for fundraisers' to begin. On one side of the wall are an array of high tech publicity materials on perspex panels which cover the walls of entrance. Here, spanning the length of one side of the wall, approximately 10 metres, are photographic representations of a number of bodies. They are recognisably female, include the bodies of both young and old, but they are not in any way visibly ill or 'cancerous'. More significantly they are mapped and criss-crossed with superimposed geometrical lines and computer generated patterns of DNA or chromosomal structures, along with attendant explanations about what science is or will uncover knowledge about the inner workings of the body. Situated in the centre of these sparkling panels is what is known as 'the challenger's wall'. This six foot plaque is strikingly noticeable at the entrance to the organisation's research centre. This is not only because of its mirror like glass appearance, but also because in contrast to other visual displays, it is densely scripted with small writing. Closer inspection reveals that there are in fact thousands of names listed. Later I learn that the names chosen by fundraisers are those who have raised over a 1000 pounds for the charity. The group of fundraisers I am with appear to naturally gravitate to the wall, picking out the names that they recognised and hovering there for some time. Some are standing in silence clasping the hands of friends or relatives who had come with them. After the visit one woman talks about her experience of visiting the research centre for the first time and seeing as she put it 'the names on the wall', saying 'I was just so in awe of it, I couldn't take it in, it was so upsetting standing there in front of my mother's name and it just sort of really threw me'.

The rapid growth of the breast cancer research charity that I have been working with since early 1999 has been striking, tied closely to the expansion, growth and diversification of breast cancer activism in the UK over the last 10 years. This is partly reflected in the demographic constitution of the organisation. Although many other charitable bodies are predominantly supported by women, market research suggests that this is even more marked in this case with over 90 per cent of supporters being female and more than half under 45. A gendered ethos about the importance of raising awareness of the disease is certainly an element in the way the charity has succeeded in mobilising support for research focused exclusively on breast cancer. Moreover even though it is partnered with a larger cancer institute and has received support and backing from a range of corporations and even pharmaceuticals, its identity as a 'grass roots' organisation, is particularly notable. This has led to a fairly rapid expansion enabling it to become a national organisation with numerous fundraising branches across the country and meeting the target of raising £15 million to build the first dedicated breast cancer research centre within the space of 10 years.

But it is distinctive in other ways, not only because it has been mainly focused on research as opposed to care or support for those with breast cancer but also because of the kind of research it funds. This is ostensibly basic science research focusing on the 'molecular pathways' thought to be associated with the development breast cancer. Notably the founding of the charity and its growth coincided with the discovery of the BRCA genes in the mid-1990s, with the official opening of the charity's research centre in 1999 taking place six months prior to the announcement of the first draft of the Human Genome. In fact at the time of my research in late 1999 more than half of the charity's research teams were looking at the function of the two BRCA genes with key scientists closely involved in the work that had led to the identification of BRCA 2. The charity has a somewhat unusual place therefore in the long standing culture of charitable funded cancer research in the UK, raising millions of pounds to focus on relatively long term basic science research but with something of a gendered activist identity.

Yet the specific kind of health 'activism' articulated in the values, ethos and work of fundraising for research in this setting is revealed not simply in demographics but, as the account of the visit to the research centre outlined above suggests, also in the way those who fundraise or support the organisation articulate their involvement. The following excerpt is a summarised account of how one woman in her late thirties told me how she came to be a fundraiser for the charity:

Anne: It was my sister-in-law that introduced me to the charity. She lived in Birmingham and sent me a Christmas card with their logo on it. She had

had breast cancer and had a mastectomy in her 40s. We went up to hers one Christmas. I said I loved the card and I said 'what's this organisation' and she said 'they're a charity and they do a £1000 challenge, why don't you have a go?' ... she was very inspirational. I went home and got my sisters and friends round with a bottle of wine. We said we would do a ball and would sink or swim on the first occasion. We organised the ball, that took about 10 months. That was my initiation ceremony. We raised £7000 first off and so exceeded all our expectations. After that Louise died. The ball was in October and Louise died in the February. She was only 44. Going to her funeral and seeing her daughters so devastated had a profound effect. I didn't do anything more for a while and then we moved house and I found some letters from Louise. One was a lovely thank you after the ball and saying that it may be too late for her but for her daughters' sake please keep fighting because research is the only way forward.

Such narratives, which were not untypical in my discussions with the charity's supporters, provide some evidence for the kinds of involvement being constituted by the act of fundraising. Studies carried out by the organisation itself in the late 1990s also revealed that,like Anne, although some had a 'personal connection' with someone who had developed the disease, more than two thirds of fundraisers had, at this time, *not* had breast cancer themselves. In fact my research with the organisation suggested that being a fundraiser in the charity was for many tied to a practice that I have described elsewhere in terms of 'memorialisation' where remembering (mostly female) relatives and loved ones who have had or died from breast cancer, is at the root of an identification with the organisation. As the response of the visitor to the research centre in the opening excerpt illustrates, being able to give such acts a permanent expression by having a name displayed on a dedicated space *within* the recently built research centre and coming to see the 'names on the wall' is for many a powerful motivation.

It is perhaps no surprise then to find that individual and collective testimonies of involvement dominate the publicity literature of the organisation. Stories such as Anne's are a regular feature of the monthly newsletter. But in a similar way the ethical values and morality associated with fundraising as memorialisation are also evident in the marketing of fundraising campaigns. For instance in one campaigning leaflet is an advert for ways of leaving a legacy for the charity in a will. The image shows two hands, one a young child, the other older, accompanied by the following text; 'the most precious thing I can leave my granddaughter is the hope of a cure for breast cancer'. On the other side of the advert is information for participating in an annual national fundraising event for the charity, alongside the following text: 'mothers' day is a celebration of the lives of the women who are closest to us, and an opportunity to remember those who have lost their lives to breast cancer'.

The particular character of breast cancer activism in this context is then sustained and reproduced in the way the organisation itself makes use of published testimony and mobilises ideas of female nurturance articulated in terms of remembrance of or hopes for past and future female relatives. In many ways such practices cannot be abstracted from and must be understood in relation to wider shifts and changes in the way breast cancer activism has and is altering the public profile of the disease (Klawiter 2000, 2004; Blackstone 2004). This has been described in terms of the increasing 'corporatisation' or 'branding' of breast cancer (King 2001) in which 'tragedy' (Fosket *et al.* 2000) and the 'moral worthiness of the breast cancer victim' is central to a public discourse about the disease (Kaufert 1998: 108; see also Saywell *et al.* 2000, and Kolker 2004). Some link this to a broader cultural trajectory in which the 'vital' suffering, pain and/or the spheres of the intimate, private or even sentimental are being increasingly and powerfully utilized across a range of public institutional arenas where issues of identity, civic participation and belonging are at stake (Berlant 1998; see also Rose and Novas 2005). In the symbiotic relationship between published narratives, campaigns and the identificatory practices of those who support the work of a cancer research charity we can see that a nexus of issues concerning the morality of intergenerational female nurturance in relation to breast cancer is an important tool in making fundraising part of a memorialising process and in reproducing this as a form of gendered health 'activism'.

Raising money in this way is however not just about witnessing loss but also in the words of fundraisers a way of 'looking forward', moving beyond the tragedy, trauma or experience of breast cancer by doing something 'positive' for future generations by funding scientific research. In fact publication of narrative and testimony in the publicity literature sits alongside 'scientific' news about the research being undertaken by the charity. Like other media, science and also some social science discourse that constituted the late years of the twentieth century, in the time before the announcement of the first draft of the human genome in 2001, the style of reporting about genetic science in the publicity literature of the charity was not immune from what has now commonly come to be understood as 'geno-hype'; a discourse that was marked by expectant and sometimes inflated rhetoric about developments in genetic knowledge and technology (Bubela and Caulfield 2004). Features of this rhetoric too were easily identifiable in how the charity communicated the work being undertaken at the research centre to its fundraisers. For instance an excerpt from a newsletter to its supporters quoted one scientist at the charity's research centre as saying:

> The centre is opening at an ideal time. A new world-wide initiative called the Human Genome Project is working to identify all the 100,000 genes that determine the way cells work in the human body.
> [...] This will be one of the most exciting events to happen in the history of medical research. (1999)

At the same time BRCA genes and other possible candidate genes were singled out as being the 'most relevant' aspects or the most significant 'major developments' in the field of breast cancer research, described in one article as 'the most important step forward since Tamoxifen was first used'. In these examples genes and genetic research were embedded within a story of hopeful or soon to be realised expertise; a discourse of 'potentiality' (Ganchoff 2004) which spoke to at the same time that it fuelled fundraisers' expectations for the science they helped fund.

For very many fundraisers I met at this time the charity's genetic research was inimical with their quest for what could be seen as 'redemptory' knowledge. This work was frequently described as 'very exciting' and 'an important way of looking towards the causes of breast cancer' and even something so otherworldly to be as one woman put it 'almost beyond the reach of the normal lay person to understand'. Although at this time in the late 1990s a minority did express some concerns about the possible 'narrowness' of a genetic approach or had worries about the implications of the current clinical application of BRCA genetics, they were still hopeful that the genetic research pursued by the charity focusing on these genes would ultimately fulfil a widespread desire and demand for scientific expertise and knowledge, positioned by most in terms of finding a 'cure' for breast cancer. This was reflected in the way one woman talked about genetic research in terms of dealing with some of the 'known' causes of breast cancer even when she didn't see such research as directly explaining or intervening in the health of her own family:

> Janice: I would hope that by identifying a gene that we would be able to find some means of intervening, it might be a drug or a test or whatever. I would like to think that there would be some way of combating the defective gene. I just think that what they are doing is excellent. It was very exciting when the team identified the BRCA2 gene … I don't think it's genetic in our family because we haven't got anyone else with breast cancer, but obviously things like the small percentage of family related, genetic breast cancers would be one of the known causes […]

Although for Janice genes didn't provide an obvious answer in understanding the breast cancers that had affected her family, she was still 'excited' by this research, which held out the hope of future treatment intervention. For some however it was precisely what was perceived as a *known* clinical application associated with new knowledge of BRCA genes which fuelled a feeling of hope and faith in the research work of the organisation. This was illustrated in what one woman said during a focus group setting in which expectations of the research being funded by the organisation were being discussed:

> Do you think it will mean there could be a fairly simple blood test for one of my daughters that could say whether she will or she won't be at risk?

Both these comments suggest that there has been a degree of enabling slippage between the activities of memorialisation for future generations through fundraising which entailed and sustained a certain degree of faith in a somewhat 'salvationary' science *and* the kinds of predictive knowledge associated with genetic testing for the BRCA genes. The way that the genetic research of the organisation could be associated with and translated into an identifiable clinical realm meant that, at least for some, the science they helped fund could be easily linked to a promissory future where predictive foreknowledge was productively linked to fundraising for future generations. This is a not an unsurprising conjunction, given that many who supported the charity often became involved after a relative had contracted the disease. It is interesting to note however how the figure of the 'BRCA carrier' sits within this nexus of interests and investments, coalescing and condensing a collective and gendered expression of inter-generational need, hope and risk in relation to breast cancer. The seemingly productive points of connection between fundraising as memorialisation, the quest for science as 'knowledge' or 'cure' and the value of predictive knowledge in the context of this particular arena of breast cancer activism provide some illustration of enabling scope of the distributed biosocialities linked to BRCA genetics.

There have of course been powerful alignments between publics and scientific research via the mechanism of charity throughout the course of the twentieth century, particularly in relation to cancer (Löwy 1997). This makes it important to examine the cultural character of the long standing interface between publics and science in the UK (Alsopp *et al.* 2004), especially where there is a close and productive alignment, as there appears to be in relation to cancer research charities (Austoker 1988). In this sense the institutional history and dynamics of charitably funded cancer research provide the backdrop for understanding how certain breast cancer 'activist' communities in the UK invest in a hype and hope filled genetic science. Novelty here is constituted by the particular *gendered* configuration of this meeting point and the way that *genetic* science is situated as part of a quest for 'redemptory' knowledge in the pursuit of a 'cure' for breast cancer.

It is perhaps the presence of the 'memorial wall' in the research centre which illustrates and indexes the extent to which fundraising as an act of hope is powerfully linked to the research undertaken by the charity. It is a kind of monument for the witnessing of loss, the pursuit of science *and* the hopes of a 'cure' for future generations. As the comments of the fundraiser at the beginning of this section illustrate, this makes it difficult to disentangle and locate the 'awe' experienced by one woman in seeing her mother's name on the wall for the first time from her perceptions of the science she is helping to fund. It is not just that DNA is situated here as quite literally a more robust locus for 'fragile memories' (Finkler 2000) in honouring the lives and memories of the sick or the dead but that it becomes a focus for hope filled investment. That is, much sought after individual *and* collective transformation of personal lives from tragedy or loss to hope, through involvement in the charity, is linked to the much hyped 'alchemy' of gene research actively invested and infused with hopes for a parallel transformation in scientific understanding and the treatment of breast cancer.

Although a potent and in many ways highly successful public/science meeting point, historical reflections on parallel powerful conjunctions between publics and the pursuit of science suggests that these are not always uniform or necessarily stable junctures (Epstein 1996). While genetic research appears to have helped fuel this kind of 'activist' identity or mode of identification within a cancer research charity for most, significantly, this is not the case for all fundraisers. In fact during the time of my research with the charity it became increasingly clear that the currently limited clinical application of BRCA genes did not sit easily with such a goal, as the quest for genes that linked the work of the charity with the Human Genome Project in earlier years became increasingly replaced by the messier business of functional genomics: a shifting context for the pursuit of genetic knowledge explored in relation to a second ethnographic excerpt.

Post-genomic complexity: silence and uncertainty

It is Autumn 2000 and the yearly national rally of the regional fundraising groups organised by the charity is taking place at a country house in central England; a suitably auspicious setting for such an event which is also an opportunity to thank fundraisers and provide them with renewed enthusiasm for future money generating ventures. It is the final day of the meeting and after a morning of presentations by the head of the fundraising section of the charity who recounts with great enthusiasm the successful official opening of the research centre there is a rather mundane discussion of health and safety issues during fundraising events. After this, what appeared to be required at the end of the weekend was a rallying and resounding endorsement about the research work the charity is undertaking. The closing speech of the day, billed as the 'Past and Future of Breast Cancer Research', at the very least held out this promise. The talk starts with an explanation about how the research strategy is focusing on the 'causes' of breast cancer. The speaker (a member of the research services team) initially points out that historically what has been thought to cause breast cancer has changed dramatically. For the next 15 minutes he examines the different ways that this has been understood and how treatments have been linked to these changing beliefs and knowledge. He plots what seems like a linear historical trajectory. This includes earlier notions that breast cancer was caused by 'black bile in the body' which has to be 'purged', to the idea that breast cancer is a 'local disease' that has to be 'cut out', interspersing his talk with fairly graphic black and white drawings of eighteenth century practitioners undertaking mastectomies. He then moves onto more recent notions of breast cancer as a disease of cells that can be treated with chemicals or radiation, but is careful to point out the 'timelag' between knowing that radiotherapy could be an affective agent, to developing a suitable means of administering this as treatment. Reaching the 1970s and the period of rapid generation of molecular knowledge, he explains how the focus is now towards what is glossed as the 'mechanism of the cells and genes'. It is only in the closing moments of his presentation that the work at the research centre is mentioned, glossed in a fairly cursory way with little discussion of the projects taking place. On reaching the end of his presentation instead of expanding on the kind of results that such research will generate, he poses a more cautionary rhetorical question. 'Does more research mean less breast cancer? Well not necessarily he says'. Without being specific he points out that current knowledge about genes and breast cancer is 'not likely to impact on patients very much as yet'. It is a remark which seems to highlight rather than discreetly pass over the gap created by the silence in this talk about anything to do with developments surrounding the BRCA genes and the translation of this newly acquired molecular knowledge into clinical care.

Talking with fundraisers after this event it was evident that they had felt somewhat disappointed. A bit 'breast cancer as it used to be' as one person put it. Another pointed out how she hadn't necessarily wanted to hear about history of surgery and left feeling a bit 'flat' because there was nothing as she said about 'what was happening in the research now' adding that 'the year before it had all been so enthusiastic'.

If the redemptory hope of genetic knowledge tied in the formative years of the charity to the hype associated with efforts to sequence the human genome had fuelled at the same time it was informed by a mode health activism situated in terms of fundraising as memorialisation, the months and years that followed which witnessed shifts in scientific understanding about how genetic knowledge would inform health care, raised questions about how this powerful conjunction between science and activism would be sustained. This issue was compounded by renewed public and media interest focused increasingly on new and troubling questions of gene patents, the use of genetic testing for insurance purposes and on-going fascination and horror in many areas of the press with the 'risk' of family history of breast cancer and dilemmas facing those identified as carriers of a mutated copy of a BRCA gene.[3] The presentation of genetic research at the rally, its deliberate lack of hype must to some extent be seen as a response to these developments. Talking to the person who had given the talk at this event several months later I asked him why he had chosen to present his speech about research in the way that he had. Initially surprised by my question he said:

Well, the specific point that just because there is more research doesn't mean there is less breast cancer has been made by a number of cancer charities. For example when we [the charity] talk about breast cancer now, we talk about 'reducing the fear', as opposed to 'eradicating' it, which used to be our old mission statement. It's changed because it's not necessarily clear how you can eradicate breast cancer, I don't know whether anyone knows whether you can stop it happening [...] the research is still just getting going and it may take a long time to really make a difference.

His comments suggested that there was an awareness within the charity of the on-going challenges of post-genomic knowledge and the need to maintain and mobilise support as well as understanding for research which, it was increasingly recognised, would be long term and vastly more complicated than previously thought. The need for a less 'hyped' presentation of genetic research, evident at the rally, was also reflected in comments which began to appear at this time in the newsletter and other publications within the charity. For instance in an article entitled 'the importance of gene research in breast cancer' to mark the tenth year of the charity's existence in 2001, an upbeat narrative about the 'pioneering research' being done at the centre is linked to another more cautionary message as this excerpt suggests:

> The last decade has seen a revolution in our understanding of what cancer is and how it progresses, although big improvements in treatments have not come as quickly as we would like. [...] The widely publicised announcement of the first draft of the human genome is an indication of the progress that has been made – however even the completion of this enormous task is just a first step in understanding how genes function, and how defects in specific genes can lead to cancer.

The dual message embedded in this excerpt concerning hope and caution suggests that defining a post-genomic space has been particularly challenging in the context of the charity. As I've explored elsewhere (see Gibbon 2007) this did in fact lead to a particular silence in the publicity literature of the charity after 2000, about the emerging field of predictive medicine associated with the BRCA genes; a lacuna which stood in contrast with the hype and hope of an earlier era of genomic 'discoveries' linked to the BRCA genes.[4]

The difficulty of fitting the complex field of post-genomic knowledge associated with BRCA genetics within the public/science dynamics that subsume the social relations of the charity was also apparent in another illustration from the fieldwork that I undertook at this time. The excerpt outlined below highlights an exchange that took place between fundraisers and scientists at the end of a routine visit of the former group of persons to the laboratories at the research centre.

During the course of the 15 months' fieldwork that I undertook with the organisation, this event was routinely characterised by a series of 'awe' filled displays in which a number of disparate objects or technologies were shown performing or being used in different experiments, often with little overall explanation about the science being undertaken. Nevertheless the end of the tours were slightly differently constituted. The 'show lab' as it was called, although at the time devoid of working scientists, brought together a number of objects whose linear juxtaposition conveyed a visual trajectory about the progress and application of molecular knowledge associated with breast cancer. Closest to the door was a mammogram or X-ray picture showing, for the first time on the tour itself, a readily identifiable outline of a breast with a compact white dot in the centre indicative of a cancerous lump; an image which has now become a widespread visual representation of breast cancer. Next to this were several brightly coloured and enlarged cytology slides of normal and cancerous breast cells with a PCR machine and a computer screen at the end of the bench. Scientists nearly always moved quickly past these two sets of objects, their hesitancy in relation to these objects displaced by open excitement as they moved towards the other objects and talked in animated ways about 'seeing' the mutations in the gene, indicated, they pointed out to fundraisers, by the gaps in the sequence of letters. Nevertheless the appearance of more familiar images such as the mammogram coupled with the linear narrative that was suggested between basic research and clinical practice through the juxtaposition of these particular objects, also seemed to prompt a series of difficult questions.

Scientists' responses differed to common variants of the question that was most often raised by fundraisers at this point in the tour, 'what good is it to know about these letters?' Many answered quickly before recourse to a scientific understanding which reflected a less than linear relationship between molecular research and clinical application. One scientist making an initial reference to the human genome project, said that knowing these genetic sequences would make it possible to 'compare normal and abnormal DNA'. Pausing for reflection he quickly added that, 'of course normal DNA would have some mutations in it anyway, so the comparison wouldn't be that clear cut.' Another scientist made a somewhat off-hand comment, in response to a more specific question about 'what exactly the benefits are of having identified the two BRACA genes', before making more uneasy efforts to backtrack on his answer:

> Well, it would be important for a woman to find out if she definitely had a BRCA mutation by having a genetic test because then she might want to have a prophylactic mastectomy … of course she might not have inherited the mutation even if it was present in other family members, in which case she wouldn't develop breast cancer and of course the actions of genes are quite complex. In fact we don't really know what BRCA2 does yet.

The kind of exchanges that took place in this setting show how during these events the contingency of the present came rushing up to meet the scientists, who in their responses appeared singularly unprepared to meet these demanding and currently unanswerable issues about the use and utility of genetic knowledge. But in thinking too about the broad terrain of biosocialities that characterise social relations in a breast cancer research charity this exchange illustrates how reference to the BRCA genes, while a resource in the hype filled years of the late 1990s, in the context of later post-genomic complexity could also be a less enabling representational source. In this context the needs, rights and vulnerabilities linked to the figure of the BRCA 'carrier' segues with a growing sense of uncertainty and complexity. The somewhat desperate recourse, by the scientists, to the limited clinical interventions available for those identified at genetic risk serves in this instance to compound and reaffirm the terrain of genomic knowledge as contingent. In this sense the encounter seems emblematic of how in a post-genomic era the image of the BRCA carrier is a representation which 'loops' back, not only as a mechanism through which enabling identification can be forged, but also as a locus from which difficult questions about the value of molecular research in pursuit of a 'cure' for breast cancer can arise.

BRCA 'eclipsed'?: systems biology and the gendered commons

This third section of this chapter brings a contemporary dimension to the analysis of the kinds of bio-social entanglements that connect BRCA genes to a particular culture of breast cancer activism by reflecting on the way that genetic research is now being contextualised and framed in the relation between science, scientists and publics in this particular breast cancer research charity. This section begins like the others outlined in this chapter with an ethnographic excerpt:

It is Autumn 2005 and I have just begun a new research initiative with the charity. I am once again on a laboratory tour for fundraisers. The scale of these events is now impressive. What had before been small groups of half a dozen visitors has now expanded to over 30 with many more formal presentations, glossy brochures and handouts. Traversing the labs this time is also a different experience from the one I had 5 years previously. Cultivating a sense of wonder is in many ways still a feature of this event – the display of the effects of liquid nitrogen in its ability to freeze things in an instant, is a spectacle everyone is willing and eager to participate in. At the same time the explanations about the science being undertaken here are longer and more comprehensive, reflecting a broader range of research projects with much reference to the challenges, complexity and timescale of molecular based research. These explanations are also now more directly linked to the novel technologies being used in the lab. Whereas before it had been the PCR machine and the ability to 'see' the mutation in the BRCA gene being pumped out in a sequence of letters on a computer screen which had been the focus of the tours, today fundraisers are introduced to micro-array techniques, fluorescent tagging and so called 'gene' or 'SNIP' chips. Significantly the collective ability of these new technologies to identify, process or store 'thousands of bits of genetic information' is used now less to induce a sense of awe than to demonstrate the scale and challenge of the task confronting the scientists. During the course of the tour we are taken to a section of the lab set aside in a separate room. One of the scientists begins to explain how, launched last year, the work taking place in this room is linked to a new initiative by the charity to set up what is described as a 'cohort study', aiming to recruit up to 100,000 women into a study of the interaction between 'genes, environment and lifestyle' as part of an investigation into the 'causes' of breast cancer. The scientists describe how women volunteers agreeing to participate are asked to initially donate a blood sample and fill in a lengthy lifestyle questionnaire and will in fact have their health tracked for up to a 40-year period. The emphasis here is on the 'care' taken in processing the blood samples whilst being shown the process by which they are spun down for extraction, barcoded, placed in multicoloured test tubes for storage and study. Not surprisingly there is a great deal of interest from the fundraisers during the tours with a number of the female fundraisers I'm with asking if 'anyone' can take part as its something they would 'definitely' want to do.

The centrality of more comprehensive and complex explanations of the genetic research on events such as the laboratory tours, illustrate the extent to which a contingent post-genomic space has and is being articulated by the organisation in communicating with fundraisers about the work that it funds. Technological awe now sits alongside discussions of the lengthy timescale, challenges and likely impact of genetic research which is couched in much more cautious terminology, with an emphasis on understanding the cellular processes and pathways through which genes, as one component in the path to developing breast cancer, do or do not become expressed. There is less stress on the work being done with BRCA genes *per se*, which although still a significant focus in terms of the research being funded by the charity, is now joined by a whole range of projects. This includes a population study, where other aetiological factors apart from genes are beginning to be visibly and vocally incorporated into an agenda for research. Despite some similarities with other national 'bio-banking' initatives, it has significantly not been described in these terms but instead in relation to more standardised medical research terminology; a 'cohort study'.

The scale and speed with which this project has been launched is impressive, recruiting thousands of women who have wanted and been willing to join the study. What seems to have been harnessed by this initiative is the mobilisation of activism as a form of memorialisation in the pursuit of a unprecedented scientific resource – a repository of genetic and lifestyle information, so vitally important to understanding and intervening in the aetiology of common and complex diseases like breast cancer. It is a logical yet also potentially perhaps transformatory moment in the evolving space of charitable fundraising in the UK, which other recent bio-bank initiatives will be keen to emulate. Thinking about the changing space of bio-social entanglements at stake here and the kinds of collective identity making and emerging materialities these developments are continuing to fuel, I want to reflect here more specifically on how such a project would not have been possible without the kind of rollercoaster of hype and hope that has been associated with BRCA genes in the preceding years.

Although these particular genes are nowhere mentioned in the publicity literature for this project and genetic factors somewhat quietly discursively incorporated alongside the importance of investigating what are described as 'lifestyle' or 'hormonal' factors, there are more implicit references to the importance and significance of genetic factors. The imagery and language used in the public recruitment drives for the cohort study draws heavily on ideas and representations of inter-generational female nurturance; idioms which implicitly I would suggest link the study through visual and linguistic metaphors to the arena of BRCA genetics and the risks which have been so publicly associated with having a family history of breast cancer. More directly the memorialising work of fundraising is given here a quite literal embodied meaning through the donation of blood for research often from relationally or generationally connected persons.

The current move within the charity and across a range of other medical and research arenas concerned with different conditions to articulate a more complex field of disease aetiology in which genes are positioned as only one link in complex disease pathways has been described by Margaret Lock in terms of a process in which the gene is being 'eclipsed' (2005). I would suggest the articulation of a more complex disease aetiology in the particular ethnographic arena outlined here points less to an 'eclipse' of the gene and more to a shifting terrain in which the legacy and imprint of the hope-filled and hype-invested arena of BRCA genetics continues to be important. In particular it is the figure of the BRCA carrier which continues to have a diffuse but nevertheless on-going iconic or representational significance for the bio-socalities being sustained and reproduced in relation to these developments. It is significant in this regard that very recent initiatives within the organisation have brought BRCA genes centre stage once again with a new campaign to reduce waiting times for genetic testing. This new campaign situates the female gene carrier, still a tiny minority of the population affected by breast cancer, as a more explicit embodiment of the collective and individual rights of what might be seen as a 'gendered commons'.[5] It is a development that provides some illustration of the way that the figure of the BRCA carrier, specifically and more generally women with a family history of the disease, have in some senses become powerful images of the embodied risk that confronts 'all women', and as a result a resource for certain kinds of collective mobilisation around the disease.

Conclusion

This chapter in examining the shifting and emerging bio-socialities of BRCA genetics has taken three illustrative moments of research with an organisation that is pivotally positioned in the past and ongoing future of molecular research focused on breast cancer. Attending to the multi-representational politics (Epstein 2003) of fundraising for a breast cancer research charity as a form of gendered health activism it has examined how this is temporally linked to a field of genetic research associated with breast cancer, mapping how the representational figure of the 'BRCA carrier' is situated in each case.

In the first instance we have seen how in an earlier era an inextricable entwining of hype and hope has been and is foundational to the successful melding of fundraising as memorialisation to the pursuit of molecular research focused on the basic science of breast cancer. Cutting to a transitionary 'post-genomic' moment the chapter has also explored the need for, as well as the challenges of efforts to manage, expectations and investment in the face of what has become a vastly more complex and long term scientific endeavour. A more contemporary illustration in the third part of this chapter highlights how efforts to align a new paradigm of 'complexity' in genetic research to memorial practices are linked to and are themselves informed by changing materialities and research objects. Here locating genes has given way to mapping the complex and intersecting pathways by which genes and other aetiological agents become connected. In each case I have suggested that it is instructive to consider how an iconic representation of the female BRCA carrier is caught up with these developments and how as an embodied image of collective and individual need(s), right(s), hope(s) or risk(s) this figure moves in enabling and also sometimes less productive ways across this temporal terrain.

In providing a sense of the shifts in these kinds of biosocial alignments formed and forming in pre and post genomic contexts I hope I have illustrated the need for social science engagement with the biosocialities of BRCA genetics in a broader frame of reference that extends beyond the clinical interface. This means addressing not only the historical and in this case gendered specificity of institutional arenas for scientific research and charitable fundraising for diseases like cancer, but also understanding the disjunctured and uneven landscape in which emergent genetic knowledge and technology is sustained and reproduced. It also includes examining how, as Landzelius and Dumit put it, the 'proxy suffering' (2006) of those affected, if not always in this instance afflicted, by breast cancer powerfully connects an articulation of individual and collective identities to the pursuit of scientific research; a configuration in which the representational figure of the BRCA carrier has in this instance become powerfully embedded.

Conclusions are premature in this instance given the fact that the 'activist' community' being sought and sustained has yet to be stabilised and is in fact itself shifting, following the recent merger with another national breast cancer advocacy organisation, and when a new paradigm for genetic research linked to micro-array techniques and long term population studies is itself only just beginning to be articulated. Importantly the 'names' being remembered and listed in the hope of better futures within the charity now extend ever closer to the science, beyond the reception of the research centre, onto new second and third memorial walls inside the laboratory corridors. But judgement will have to be reserved for the time being on whether this and the practices and processes explored in this chapter index an emergent social form that can articulate the sort of 'civic science' some argue is demanded and made possible by a new paradigm of 'systems biology' taking shape across a range of genomic research arenas (Fortun and Fortun 2005). The stakes are high for all concerned, requiring attentiveness to the real opportunities and on-going dangers of the diverse and evolving bio-social entanglements between the pursuit of scientific knowledge and breast cancer activism.

Acknowledgements

Sections of this chapter are amended from *Breast Cancer Genes and the Gendering of Knowledge. Science and Citizenship in the Cultural Context of the 'New' Genetics,* (2007) by Sahra Gibbon. Reproduced by permission of Palgrave Macmillan.

Notes

1   Recent published figures in relation to a number of high profile reports and assessments in the UK, point to the need for this broader perspective which suggests

that relatively few numbers of women have been positively identified as gene carriers (approximately 1,500) with carrier status remaining something of unknown entity for the vast majority seen in specialist cancer genetic clinics for some time to come (see for instance NICE 2004).The disparities between the number of women being referred and those being identified as carriers must be situated in relation to technological limitations, economic costs or timescale of mutation screening or predictive testing, as well the currently unknown numbers of women who choose not to undertake these interventions or who simply refuse to be recruited into predictive practices in the first place.

2 Some aspects of my research have explored this more distributed domain of identity formation and knowledge practices in clinical settings see (Gibbon 2007).

3 See for instance 'US Firm double costs of UK cancer checks', *The Guardian*, 17 January 2000 or 'MPs slam insurers on genes', *The Guardian*, May 2001.

4 There was, however, in some of this literature a higher profile given to discussing one of the first drugs for the treatment of breast cancer to be developed from molecular based knowledge, Herceptin.

5 This concept borrows from Marilyn Strathern's discussion of how ideas of 'community' and 'the commons' have been mobilised in pursuit of accountability in relation to a range of initiatives surrounding genomics in the UK (2004).

References

Allsop, J., Jones, K. and Baggott, R. (2004) 'Health consumer groups in the UK: a new social movement?', *Sociology of Health and Illness*, 26(6): 737–56.

Anglin, M.K. (1997)'Working from the inside out; implications of breast cancer activism for bio-medical policies and practices', *Social Science and Medicine*, 44(9): 1043–415.

Austoker, J. (1988) *A History of the Imperial Cancer Research Fund 1902–1986*, Oxford: Oxford University Press.

Berlant, L. (ed.) (1998) 'Intimacy: a special issue', *Critical Inquiry*, Winter.

Blackstone, A. (2004) '"It's just about being fair" activism and the politics of volunteering in the breast cancer movement', *Gender and Society*, 18(3), June: 350–68.

Bubela, T.M and Caulfields, T. (2004) 'Do the print media "hype" genetic research? A comparison of newspaper stories and peer-reviewed research', *CMAJ*, 170(9): 1399–407.

Callon, M. and Rabeharisoa, V. (2003) '"Research in the wild" and the shaping of new social identities', *Technology in Society*, 25(2): 193–204.

Cartwright, L. (2000) 'Community and the public body in breast cancer activism', in Marschessault, J. and Sawchuck, K. (eds) *Wild Science: Reading Feminism, Medicine and the Media*, New York: Routledge, pp. 120–38.

D'Agincourt-Canning, L. (2001) 'Experiences of genetic risk: disclosure and the gendering of responsibility', *Bioethics*, 15(3): 231–47.

Epstein, S. (2003) 'Inclusion, diversity, and biomedical knowledge-making: the multiple politics of representation', in Oudshoorn, N. and Pinch, T. (eds) *How Users Matter: The Co-Construction of Users and Technology*, Boston, MA: MIT Press.

Epstein, S. (2007) 'Patient groups and health movements', in Hackett, E.J., Amsterdamska, O., Lynch, M. and Wacjman, J. (eds) *New Handbook of Science and Technology Studies*, Cambridge, MA: MIT Press.

Finkler, K (2000) 'The kin in the gene: the medicalization of family and kinship in American society' in *Current Anthropology*, 42(2): 235–83.

Fortun, K. and Fortun, M. (2005) 'Scientific imaginaries and ethical plateaus', *Contemporary U.S. toxicology*, 107(1): 43–54.

Fosket, J. (2004) 'Constructing "high-risk women": the development and standardization of a breast cancer risk assessment tool', *Science, Technology and Human Values*, 29(3), Summer: 291–313.

Fosket, J., Ruth, J., Karran, A. and LaFia, C. (2000) 'Breast cancer in popular women's magazines from 1913–1997', in Ferguns, S.J. and Kasper, A.S. (eds) *Breast Cancer: Society Constructs an Epidemic*, New York: St Martin's Press.

Franklin, S., Lury, C. and Stacey, J. (2000) *Global Nature, Global Culture*, London: Sage Publications.

Ganchoff, C. (2004) 'Regenerating movements: embryonic stem cells and the politics of potentiality', *Sociology of Health and Illness*, 26(6): 757–74.

Gibbon, S. (2007) *Breast Cancer Genes and the Gendering of Knowledge: Science and Citizenship in the Cultural Context of the 'New' Genetics*, Basingstoke: Palgrave Macmillan.

Hacking, I. (1986) 'Making up people', in Weller *et al.* (eds) *Re-consctructing Individualism: Autonomy, Individualism and the Self in Western Thought,* Stanford, CA: Stanford University Press.

Hallowell, N. (1999) 'Doing the right thing: genetic risk and responsibility', in Conrad, P. and Gabe, J. (eds) *Sociological Perspective on the New Genetics*, Oxford: Blackwell Publishers, pp. 97–120.

Heath, D., Rapp, R. and Taussig, K. (2003) 'Genetic citizenship', in Night, D. and Vincent, J. (eds) *A Companion to the Anthropology of Politics*, Oxford: Blackwell Publishing.

Henderson, L. and Kitzinger, J. (1999) 'The human drama of genetics: "hard" and "soft" media representations of inherited breast cancer', in Conrad, P. and Gabe, J. (eds) *Sociological Perspectives on the New Genetics*, Oxford: Blackwell Publishers, pp. 59–78.

Kaufert, P. (1996) 'Women and the debate over mammography: an economic, political, and moral history', in Sargents, C.F. and Brettell, C.B. (eds) *Gender and Health: An International Perspective*, Upper Saddle River, NJ: Prentice-Hall, pp. 167–86.

Kaufert, P. (1998) 'Women, resistance and the breast cancer movement', in Lock, M. and Kaufert, P. (eds) *Pragmatic Women and Body Politics*, Cambridge: Cambridge University Press, pp. 287–309.

Kaufert, P. (2003) 'From the lab to the clinic: the story of genetic testing for hereditary breast cancer', *Head, Heart and Hand: Partnerships for Women's Health in Canadian Environments*, Vol. 1.1, Toronto National Network on Environment and Women's Health, pp. 487–506.

King, S. (2001) 'An all-consuming cause: breast cancer, corporate philanthropy, and the market for generosity', *Social Text*, 19: 115–43.

Klawiter, M. (2000) 'From private stigma to global assembly: transforming the terrain of breast cancer', in Burawoy, M. Blum, J.A., Zsuszsa Gille, S.G., Gowan, T., Haney, L., Klawiter, M., Steven H. Lopez, S.H., Riain, S., O., and Thayer, M. (eds) *Global Ethnography: Forces, Connections and Imaginations in a Postmodern World*, Berkeley, CA: University of California Press, pp. 299–334.

Klawiter, M. (2004) 'Breast cancer in two regimes: the impact of social movements on illness experience', *Sociology of Health and Illness*, 26(6): 845–74.

Kolker, E. (2004) 'Framing as a cultural resource in health social movements: funding activism and the breast cancer movement in the US 1990–1993', in Brown, P. and

Zavestoski, S. (eds) *Social Movements in Health,* Sociology of Health and Illness Monographs, Oxford: Blackwell Publishing, pp. 820–44.

Konrad, M. (2005) *Narrating the New Predictive Genetics: Ethics, Ethnography and Science*, Cambridge: Cambridge University Press.

Landzelius, K. and Dumit, J. (2006) 'Introduction', Special theme issue: patient organization movements, *Social Science and Medicine*, February: 529–82.

Lantz, P. and Booth, K. (1998) 'The social construction of the breast cancer epidemic', *Social Science and Medicine*, 46(7): 907–18.

Lerner, B.H. (2003) *The Breast Cancer Wars: Hope, Fear and the Pursuit of a Cure in Twentieth-Century America*, New York: Oxford University Press.

Lock, M. (2005) 'The eclipse of the gene and the return of divination', *Current Anthropology*, 46, Supplement, December: S47–S70.

Löwy, I. (1997) *Between Bench and Bedside: Science, Healing and Interleukin-2 in a Cancer Ward*, Cambridge, MA: Harvard University Press.

Montini, T. (1996) 'Gender and emotion in the advocacy for breast cancer informed consent legislation', *Gender and Society*, 10(1): 9–23.

NICE (National Institute of Clinical Excellence) and NCCPC (National Collaborating Centre for Primary Care (2004) 'Familial breast cancer: the classification and care of women at risk of familial breast cancer in primary, secondary and tertiary care', http://www.nice.org.uk/.

Parthasarathy, S. (2003) 'Knowledge is power: genetic testing for breast cancer and patient activism in the United States and Britain', in Oudshoorn, N. and Pinch, T. (eds) *How Users Matter: The Co-Construction of Users and Technology*, Cambridge, MA and London: MIT Press.

Potts, L. (ed.) (2000) *Ideologies of Breast Cancer*, London: Macmillan.

Rabinow, P. (1996) 'Artificiality and enlightenment: from socio-biology to bio-sociality', in Rabinow, P. (ed.) *Essays on the Anthropology of Reason*, Princeton, NJ: Princeton University Press, pp. 91–112.

Rapp, R. (1999) *Testing Women, Testing the Fetus: The Social Impact of Amniocentesis in America*, New York: Routledge.

Rose, N. and Novas, C. (2005) 'Biological Citizenship' in Ong, A. and Collier, S.J. (eds) *Global Assemblages: Technology, Politics, and Ethics as Anthropological Problems*, Malden, MA: Blackwell, pp. 439–64.

Saywell, C., Beattie, L. and Henderson, L. (2000) 'Sexualised illness: the newsworthy body in media representations of breast cancer', in Potts, L. (ed.) *Ideologies of Breast Cancer*, London: Macmillan, pp. 37– 62.

Strathern, M. (2004) *Commons and Borderlands: Working Papers on Interdisciplinarity, Accountability and the Flow of Knowledge*, Wantage: Sean Kingston Publishing.

Wonderling, D., Hopwood, P., Cull, A., Douglas, F., Watson, M., Burn, J. and McPherson, K. (2001) 'A descriptive study of UK cancer genetics services: an emerging clinical response to the new genetics', *British Journal of Cancer*, 85(2): 166–70.

Zavestoski, S., McCormick, S. and Brown, P. (2004) '"Gender, embodiment and disease: environmental breast cancer activists" challenges to science, the bio-medical model and policy', *Science as Culture*, 13(4): 563–86.

2 Brains, pedigrees, and promises

Lessons from the politics of autism genetics

Chloe Silverman

Patricia Stacey is a memoirist who attributes her son's recovery from the threat of autism to "floor time," an intensive program of early behavioral intervention. One of the many explanatory narratives that circulate in parent and research communities devoted to the autism spectrum disorders proposes that seemingly unaffected parents exhibit, in milder form, the behaviors and sensitivities of their children. So when Stacey describes how a therapist's passing comment about her tendency to "space out" during sessions with her son led her to recognize her own sensory intolerances and defensiveness, she is speaking to a community that will make rapid sense of the genetic claims that ground her observation. Her son's therapist made her recognize that "[s]ometimes the children we are working with are just exaggerated versions of their parents" (Stacey 2003: 254). For Stacey, this meant that the "developmental, individual-difference, relationship-based model," a program of "interactive play" (Wieder and Greenspan 2003) that fosters the ability to sustain interpersonal interactions that is often absent in children diagnosed with autism, simultaneously healed her son and altered her perception of herself. Treating her son changed her understanding of her own fragile sensory tolerances, so that when she sought to shape her son's development, she did so from the perspective of a semi-insider, one who also felt assaulted by the barrage of sights and sounds in her environment.

To explain her experience, Stacey writes, "As geneticists study autism, they are discovering that autism isn't merely passed down by people with a diagnosis, but it is also passed down by parents with a few autistic characteristics. Geneticists call people who do not fit into all the diagnostic criteria 'broad autistic phenotypes'" (Stacey 2003: 255), a characterization that allows researchers to take account of nominally typical relatives in genetic studies (Dawson *et al.* 2002). Autism is not always a severe disorder, but occurs in milder forms shading into normality. Stacey continues:

> Time and again when I have been talking to women with children with autism, I hear a resonant story. I heard nearly the same story twice from two different mothers who had never met. The couple goes to a lecture on autism or visits a therapist shortly after their child receives a diagnosis. The couple learns that people with autism have systematic minds, like things in certain orders, have

trouble with transitions – that people with autism are not social – that they may be good with math and music, or they are highly visual. The husband walks out of the classroom, or office, and says, "My God, they've just been describing me."

(Stacey 2003: 255)

That shock of recognition arises from a particular story about the heritability and genetic nature of a diagnostic category that has been rendered relatively stable through the production of standardized behavioral screening tools, in addition to an entry in the *Diagnostic and Statistical Manual of Mental Disorders*. Although there are no biological markers for autism, pediatricians know that when a child comes into their office with a developmental delay, they should look for "qualitative impairment" in social, communicative, and behavioral domains with onset before the age of three for "full spectrum" autism, and a similar set of traits with present (though perhaps atypical) language in Asperger Syndrome, a related disorder (APA 2000). Those descriptions of traits were first assembled and used to define a specific syndrome by Leo Kanner in 1943 and Hans Asperger in 1944 (Kanner 1943; Asperger 1944 [1991]). Asperger's cases, drawn from a clinic in Austria, used language, while most of Kanner's children did not speak or only echoed words and phrases. The two researchers, who were not aware of each other's work at the time, described children who were as uniquely alike as a category in their "extreme autistic aloneness" and "insistence on sameness" (Kanner 1943) as they were different in the specifics of their individual fixations and private language.

These lists of diagnostic traits have come to ground two very different discourses of kinship in the world of autism research. Autistic behaviors support claims for kinship based on likeness across groups of people with autism, and claims based on familial tendencies. Both claims are increasingly, though not exclusively, framed in the language of genetics. Rayna Rapp and Faye Ginsburg have argued for the centrality of kinship narratives in changing the social and legal realities of disability, emphasizing "the cultural work performed by the circulation of kinship narratives through various public media as an essential element in the refiguring of the body politic as envisioned by advocates of both disability and reproductive rights" (Rapp and Ginsburg 2001: 535). Hence, the meaning of kinship for these groups extends beyond the descriptive. Claims of kinship form the basis for discourses of affective entitlement. Shared genes become a way of talking about affection, love, community, and innate understanding. They act as proxies for these other ideas because spokespersons and relatives of people with autism work in a landscape shaped by the historical legacies of autism research.

Autism has become genetic (Silverman and Herbert 2003), but it has become so in the wake of a long history of theorizing about autism as a form of organic emotional deficit in those diagnosed, or as caused by an emotional deviance in their parents, where "the precipitating factor in infantile autism is the parent's wish that the child should not exist" (Bettelheim 1967: 125). Autism has been about failures of love, disorders of affect. The act of speaking for people with autism is legitimated by multiple affinities built on genetic association and physiological likeness, or by the idea of heritability and the affective claims of parenthood. Affect works as a vocabulary of motivation; it describes practices by placing them firmly within the world of human relationships without reducing those relationships to material investments.

Paul Rabinow's concept of biosociality opened up a particularly fertile space for social scientists to explore the implications of genetic and genomic technologies (Rabinow 1996a, 1996b). Where Rabinow suggested that with biosociality "a truly new type of autoproduction will emerge," where our increased ability to alter genomes will lead to a moment when "[n]ature will be remade through technique and will finally become artificial, just as culture becomes natural," contemporary versions of genomics often emphasize the genetic consequences of unintentional acts rather than "technique" (Rabinow 1996b: 99). They return to older discourses of genetics, heredity, and kinship. As genetic technologies fail to yield the comprehensive knowledge that has been promised by their promoters, theories and rhetorics of miscegenation, eugenics, atavism and degeneration return to haunt genetic discourse and the communities that are built around genetic knowledge. Likewise, explanatory narratives supplement genetic discourses with concepts from kinship, physiology, and psychiatry. These discourses are evident in reports of "assortative mating" when two behaviorally similar humans (two computer geeks, two engineers) decide to marry and have children with a higher likelihood of developing autism (Baron-Cohen 2003), or parent activists unified by the idea that childhood immunizations in combination with a genetic inability to metabolize toxic substances "triggered" their children's autism (Kirby 2005).

Rabinow imagined an array of "pastoral keepers" to help groups defined by shared genetic disorders understand their fate: "Fate it will be. It will carry no depth. It makes absolutely no sense to seek the meaning of the lack of a guanine base because it has no meaning" (Rabinow 1996b: 102). But for complex disorders like autism, where establishing the reality of the "genetic" nature of the disorder requires ongoing social, emotional and especially discursive work, meaning-making practices are almost everywhere you look. "Pastoral keepers," if they offer behavioral therapies, nutritional supplements, or counseling, do so not merely in order to inform, but also to direct and shape. Uta Frith, an expert on the cognitive psychology of Asperger Syndrome, addresses people with Asperger Syndrome directly, emphasizing her opinion of the importance of recognizing that they are far from normal, despite temptations to regard the disorder as a "normal personality variant". "Presumed normality does not make allowance for sudden gaps in the carefully woven fabric of compensatory learning … It is not easy, but in controlling themselves they are dealing with the one person over whom they rightly have power" (Frith 1991: 23–4). Frith's statement, made with the full force of her considerable experience, combines a judgment of the cognitive abnormality of people with Asperger Syndrome with a recommendation about normative behavior: they will have to adjust.

Other scholars have joined Rabinow in considering the consequences of identities based on biological facts, facts which, if socially constituted, still take shape in ways that are unruly and capable of upsetting established categories of pathology and normality. In keeping with these recent writings on "biosociality," "genetic citizenship," and "biological citizenship" (Rabinow 1996b; Rapp 1999; Rose and Novas 2003), this chapter explores the politics and economies enabled by the biological knowledge and social practices which work to construct and stabilize self-conscious populations. Ian Hacking has suggested that autism might be a case of what he calls "dynamic nominalism," the process through which expert descriptions and the independent actions of the populations that they define work together to produce new identities in a kind of "looping effect" (Hacking 2000, 2006). For Hacking, autism is a syndrome of this historical moment, its fabled increase in prevalence a product of improved surveillance and the adoption of the identity by parents for their children and by individuals for themselves – even in the absence of an identified genetic "cause." Hacking's suggestions mirror those of many epidemiologists who attempt to explain the cause of the recent increase in autism diagnoses (e.g. Fombonne 2001; Gernsbacher *et al.* 2005). There remains work to be done in establishing connections between the "life politics" of biosociality, and the "looping effects" described by Hacking – processes that in practice turn out to be closely aligned. The "making up" of genetic populations often entails the same kinds of investment and awareness on the part of the subjects of diagnosis that Hacking describes in the case of mental illnesses (Hacking 1999).

Conversely, severe disorders like autism only serve to emphasize the inescapability of identities that are shaped by diagnoses, especially when the subjects of diagnosis are children. Members of these groups see their only option as that of speaking *as* a parent of a child with autism, an autistic person, or a person with "autistic traits." What Hacking describes as "autonomous behavior" (Hacking 1999) at the level of the diagnosed population involves authority that is predicated on the ability of some to speak *for* members of a population unified under a diagnostic label. Establishing the authority of this embodied expertise is no simple operation. It involves claims of priority based on unstable narratives of genetic likeness, which sometimes translate as parenthood, sometimes pathology, and sometimes nonpathological difference. As early as 1967, Clara Claiborne Park argued for the advantages of parents' knowledge over professional observations in terms of their ability to interpret "patterns of behavior that might seem strange to an outsider but are not so to parents, who see them in their normal children as well as in the deviate, and who also recognize them in themselves" (Park 1967: 182). Parents, scientists, and self-advocates express the points of dissonance between expert and bodily or experiential knowledge as problems of affect, using the language of disappointment, heartache, exclusion, and mourning. Studying the testimony that affect enables and affectively mediated practices of membership and exclusion can provide insight into the practices that connect expert knowledge and the production of individual or collective identities.

In order to show how this works, I describe two cases. First, I consider a contemporary set of institutional formations constructed by parent groups who used their affective commitments to dispute the proper organization of research on material from populations composed of themselves and their children. Next,

I consider how self-advocates with autism and Asperger Syndrome (AS) accept a genetic and neurological definition of the syndrome but protest against the use of behavioral and sometimes medical interventions. They argue that seeking interventions reflects an unacceptable devaluation of autistic traits and tendencies that are disabilities only with respect to social barriers. Work to define autism acts as a reminder that genetic identities are only as fixed as the meanings attached to them. At one level, it is not entirely clear what it means to be, for instance, "a little autistic." At another, a general understanding of this term among researchers and increasingly in popular culture reflects a social consensus that is crucial for the shaping of identity and concepts of health, disability, and personhood. Put slightly differently, the presumed genetic status of autism grants permission for certain kinds of kinship relations (relationships of likeness between "high" and "low" functioning autistic individuals, or the recognition of similarities between parents and children), as well as expressions of emotional commitment and obligation, and it excludes others. Who gets caught up in autism becomes a question of both pragmatic and ethical consequence.

Parenthood, pedigrees, and partiality in autism genetics

In a speech to a national convention, Jon Shestack, who founded the Cure Autism Now Foundation (CAN) with his wife, Portia Iverson, spoke about fatherhood and autism, evoking histories of parent-blaming and explaining his devotion to research:

> Dov is now eleven, and I'm still trying to figure out how best to love him. All the ways they teach men to be – loud, fast, aggressive – aren't effective with an autistic kid. You come home from the office and make a big commotion, looking for a big reaction, like you're the greatest, most fun dad, but that's just not going [to] get you any closer. They say autistic kids don't imitate very well, but their parents imitate quite well and after a couple of years of non-responsiveness sometimes you just sort of check out.
>
> (CAN 2003)

For Shestack, it is easier to express his commitment to his son through his work as an advocate: "That's what I know how to do for Dov. That's how I know best to love him" (CAN 2003).

Genetics operates as a resource for parent advocacy organizations. It gives them leverage against autism researchers and helps them shorten research timelines that look sluggish to parents urgently seeking treatments for their children. CAN believes that "with enough determination, money and manpower, science can be hurried," (CAN n.d.) and for CAN, science has often meant genetics. The status of autism as "one of the most heritable complex disorders, with compelling evidence for genetic factors and little or no support for environmental influence" (Veenstra-VanderWeele and Cook 2004: 379) and the corresponding centrality of genetics in autism research were not inevitable. Early twin studies have given way to whole genome scans, but, as with other complex genetic conditions, limits to genetic explanations have been incorporated into the discourse of autism genetics in what Hedgecoe (2001) has called a "narrative of enlightened geneticization." Another discourse of heredity, the language of parenthood and family ties, provides a resource of a more affective sort – although both are responses and alternatives to earlier psychogenic theories of autism.

Up until 2006, the two major research-related autism organizations were the Cure Autism Now Foundation (CAN) and the National Alliance for Autism Research (NAAR). They were founded almost simultaneously, on opposite coasts: NAAR in New Jersey in 1994, and CAN in California in 1995. Both organizations have committed millions to autism research over the past decade.[1] Both organizations also understand that their status as parent groups lends a particular perspective to research, and both groups incorporate parents into the grant review process.[2] More importantly, both groups have made use of the status of their members as parents to influence the direction and stakes of genetics research in autism. For these groups, genetics becomes the means to repair broken families as much as it is a sign of familial likeness.

The founders of CAN, Portia Iverson and Jonathan Shestack, are both involved in the Hollywood film and television industries. Iverson has won awards for her work in television; Shestack has worked as a producer. Their son, Dov, was diagnosed shortly before Iverson and Shestack founded CAN in 1995. Shestack and Iverson decided to reform the practice of genetics research in autism by leveraging their control over genetic materials and the social networks of parent communities. This technique is not unique to CAN or NAAR. Rather, it is one of the strategies used by groups that are personally invested in the outcomes of scientific research. Steven Epstein has demonstrated that AIDS treatment activists used many of the same strategies, including establishing themselves as "representatives" for their community and drawing explicit connections between political and ethical arguments and the design and methodology of research (Epstein 1995). What these attempts at intervention into biomedical fact production have in common are the use of tactics that go beyond the simple provision of funds to involve strategic investment and the management of material resources, with the aim of altering not only the outcomes of research, but the normative behavior of researchers (Merton 1973 [1942]). As outsiders to the world of genetics research, parents were able to demand that scientists actually adhere to the stated imperatives of "good science," despite the fact that actual scientific practice is a distinctly counternormative affair, often rife with the secrecy, concerns over reputation, and failures of skepticism that so dismayed Iverson and Shestack (Mulkay 1976).

The founding of AGRE, the Autism Genetic Resource Exchange, is one of the more visible success stories in autism research. According to most accounts, Portia Iverson and Jon Shestack met with experts in the autism research field and determined that genetics offered the most promise as an avenue of research and that effective genetic research would require DNA samples from at least 100 multiplex families (families with two or more family members with the condition). When they began contacting genetics researchers, they discovered that "[a]s as group, the scientists had collected DNA from the necessary 100 families. Individually, however, no single team had DNA from anywhere near that number. And because the teams were not sharing samples, none of them had enough DNA for a thorough study" (Zitner 2003). According to one story, the couple met with the five major researchers working on the genetics of autism, showed them a photograph of their son, reiterated the rates of autism and the possibility of rising incidence, and asked them to pool their samples in the interest of accelerating research, allowing intentional replication of findings, and avoiding overlapping investigations. The researchers refused to cooperate. Shestack explained that "[e]veryone wanted to be the first to find the genes – their careers depended on being first – and they didn't want anyone else to get a competitive advantage" (Zitner 2003).

The only solution was to control "the coin of the realm: DNA" (Zitner 2003). In 1997, Portia Iverson and Jon Shestack concluded that they would form their own gene repository, using their status as a parent organization to access and recruit families. They eventually produced a sample of over 400 multiplex families, meaning families with at least two affected siblings.[3] This came to over 800 samples from individuals with autism spectrum disorders, or over 1,000 samples including family members (Geschwind *et al.* 2001; AGRE n.d.). By the summer of 2006, the collection totaled 12,000 families (CAN 2006). The acronym for the Autism Genetic Resource Exchange, pronounced like the word "agree," makes explicit CAN's objective: to promote collaborative work on shared samples. AGRE's samples, including purified DNA, serum samples, and immortalized cell lines from all family members, are available approximately at cost to qualified researchers. Phenotypic information, obtained at home visits, is available to participant researchers via a built-to-purpose database called ISAAC (Internet System for Assessing Autistic Children), designed by the father of a child with autism. The project was funded entirely with more than $6 million in private donations, although a substantial grant from the NIMH (National Institute of Mental Health) was awarded in 2002. Significantly, and possibly in response to initiatives like AGRE, recipients of substantial NIMH grants in genetics are now required to share data and biomaterials acquired during the grant period through the NIMH repository.

CAN/AGRE chose to exploit parental networks to create a material resource in the form of a genetic repository. A genetics initiative headed by NAAR, the Autism Genetics Cooperative (AGC), used a different strategy. If AGRE tried to create something like an "an obligatory passage point" (Callon 1987) for genetics researchers, AGC incorporated the professional and social worlds of the scientists themselves, recognizing that the desire for recognition and the fear of being preempted were as significant for genetics researchers as speed and treatment targets were for parents. The founders of NAAR, like CAN, reasoned that the combined effects of the NIH funding structure, academic career trajectories and tenure considerations, and the increasing commercialization of genetic information had created a context of intense competition and secrecy. In an attempt to overcome this barrier, NAAR addressed the culture of autism genetics research, using their status as a parent organization as a tool for organizing scientific work. For NAAR, research was better organized by those with personal, indeed affective and familial, stakes in the outcome.

NAAR-AGC sought to solve the problem of collaboration by acting, in the words of one staff member, as an "honest broker" for autism geneticists. NAAR selected twenty-two international sites, which included the most experienced researchers in the field of autism genetics, with the objective of encouraging them to pool their samples and work collaboratively. Once yearly, the participant researchers attended a retreat at Calloway Gardens in Atlanta, GA. Only participant researchers were allowed and attendees were instructed to confine their discussions to autism genetics. Several ground rules set the tone for the meetings. Only unpublished work was presented during the course of the retreat, confidentiality was strictly respected, as was priority, and democratic participation was encouraged. Junior researchers participated alongside more experienced colleagues (NAAR 2004). It took about four years, but an atmosphere of trust was gradually established. NAAR fashioned itself as a virtual persona capable of possessing entirely pure motives; using this persona, representatives of NAAR were able to create a space in which collaboration might emerge. Both CAN and NAAR parlayed their identity as parent groups into a privileged position with respect to their ability to influence the social worlds of scientists. They capitalized on their social and biological role as parents by acting in the role of broker and paradoxically neutral agent, a morally pure persona who transformed emotionality into a resource. For these groups, the partiality that comes with parenthood was an asset rather than a liability. Although experts on advisory boards ensure an "objective" evaluation of proposals, parents add an essential component of affective investment.

The NAAR-Autism Genome Project (AGP), an initiative funded and supported jointly with four member institutes of the National Institutes of Health, began in 2003. The project incorporated most of the major autism genetics research networks, including AGRE, in a consortium that a press release referred to as a "collaboration of collaborations" (NAAR n.d.).[4] As of February 2007, both CAN and NAAR merged with the new and wealthier parent organization Autism Speaks (NAAR 2005a; CAN 2007). Having altered the terrain of genetics research, the genetics initiatives of CAN and NAAR were functionally combined within a single organization. Meanwhile, the language of genetics researchers working on autism has adapted to reflect the unpromising results of the multiple genome scans conducted thus far. The NAAR Autism Genome Project is clear on the matter. It is not seeking a genetic cause for autism, but is "designed to map the human genome in the search for autism susceptibility genes – the genes responsible for the inherited risk of autism" (NAAR 2005b).

Autistic biosociality: Asperger Syndrome and autistic cousins

In the fundraising appeals of organizations like CAN, NAAR, and the Autism Society of America (ASA), broken family relations are repeatedly invoked. The

ASA website features flash videos of family photographs which tear to isolate one child (ASA 2005). Even so, the genetic research programs sponsored by these organizations make use of the existence of autistic traits in direct family members. In contrast, an emerging self-advocacy movement of autistic individuals has used genetics as a basis for a different kind of appeal. For members of this group, the reality of a genetically-defined population behind the autism diagnosis is equally important, but it supports a different set of claims for representation and entitlement. The emergence of an autism self-advocacy movement has come about as a result of a resurgence of professional interest in the Asperger Syndrome diagnosis and the "broader autism spectrum" within the autism research community, on the one hand, and an already-established framework of parent organizations that allowed large-scale connections to be formed between people "on the spectrum," on the other. Some researchers speculate that fairytales about changelings are in fact records of the presence of autism in centuries past (Frith 1989), but for many parents autism is a family trait, it grants them an even stronger form of genetic kinship with their affected children, but also, and more significantly, brings those same children into relations of genetic likeness with autistic adults. If in some cases of childhood disability, experiences of kinship are disrupted by an apparent lack of visible similarity between parents and children, in autism, genetic kinship is defined *in terms* of disability (Rapp 2000). Many parents recognize autistic traits in themselves and obtain diagnoses only after their child is found to have autism (Harmon 2004a).

The description of Asperger Syndrome as an autism-like disorder with relatively unimpaired language was all but ignored in the English-speaking world until 1981, when Lorna Wing published an article arguing for its applicability and suggesting that many psychiatric patients were better described by a diagnosis of Asperger Syndrome (Frith 1991; Wing 1981), although in other countries, researchers had worked with Asperger's case descriptions for decades (Inose and Fukushima 2005).[5] Experts who approach autism from the perspective of cognitive psychology have focused on the cognitive strengths associated with autism, as well as the deficits (Frith 1989; Baron-Cohen 2003). This interest works as a resource for individuals on the autism spectrum who write about "autistic ways of knowing," suggesting that autistic abilities are not "splinter skills" but instead reflect a different and not necessarily pathological cognitive organization (Dawson *et al.* 2005). In emphasizing a pattern of strengths and weaknesses, these researchers follow Asperger's focus on the promise of the children he described. He argued that their autistic traits might be channeled into professional careers, and that "[a]ble autistic individuals can rise to eminent positions and perform with such outstanding success that one may even conclude that only such people are capable of certain achievements. It is as if they had compensatory abilities to counter-balance their deficiencies" (Asperger 1991 [1944]: 88) including their ability to focus on topics of special interest to the exclusion of all else. Although Asperger might have been moved to emphasize the cognitive strengths of his subjects because of the political climate of 1940s Austria (Frith 1991), contemporary advocates also argue that an emphasis on autistic strengths is crucial to adult success (Grandin 2004).

Even as expert interest in Asperger Syndrome may have led to an upsurge in diagnoses and self-diagnoses, new communities have blossomed independently on the Internet. One advocate suggests that "[t]he Internet is for many high functioning autistics what sign language is for the deaf," and argues for parallels between "emerging autistic culture" and the formation of the disability rights movement (most notably the Deaf community) and the psychiatric survivors movement (Dekker 1999). Others argue for parallels – and even political alliances – with the gay rights movement (Schwartz 2006). The annual Autreat, founded in 1996 by Jim Sinclair, provides a space for autistic individuals from any point on the spectrum where they are free to engage in "self stimulatory behaviors" or "stimming" that might lead to ostracism in the workplace. Promotional materials state that "[w]e do not expect you to 'act normal' or to behave like a neurotypical person at Autreat. It is perfectly acceptable at Autreat to rock, stim, echo, perseverate, and engage in other 'autistic' behaviors" (Sinclair 2005). Conference badges are color coded. Green badges invite others to initiate social interactions, red is a request to be left alone, and a yellow badge means approach if you are already acquainted. Members of the first Autreat formed the Autism Network International (ANI), a community with a distinct culture based on shared experiences of difference and the pleasure that came with being "able to communicate with someone in my own language," an experience that Sinclair refers to as "autistic first contact" (Sinclair 2005). Members of ANI, including "Aspies" and those with autism diagnoses argue for respect for their neurological differences and those of their "Autistic Cousins" (sometimes abbreviated to AC), those with language and social differences arising from sensory processing disorders or brain injuries. They freely suggest that "neurotypical" or NT perceptions and behavior are not so much normal as normative.

Advocates recall that communities of autistic adults met through Internet mailing lists originally established by parent advocacy organizations devoted to treatment (Dekker 1999; Sinclair 2005). Parents "of less-communicative autistic people" sought out "verbally proficient autistic adults," including some who had "fit descriptions of 'low functioning' autistic people" when they were younger, as interpreters for their children, sometimes going as far as to request panels of autistic adults at parent conferences (Sinclair 2005). By emphasizing kinship across the autism spectrum, adults with autism argue for their status as spokespeople and biologically ideal translators for children who may seem unlike their parents. A literal profusion of websites addressing self-advocacy have arisen, most notably neurodiversity.com ("honoring the variety of human wiring"), autistics.org and aspiesforfreedom.com. For the self-advocacy community, the desire for a cure is an unethical position that entails the denial of autistic humanity.[6] Websites feature T-shirts which note that "Not Being Able to Speak is Not the Same as Not Having Anything to Say," "I Love My Perseverations," or "Autists are People Not Puzzles" (a reference to the autism awareness ribbon produced by the

Autism Society of America).[7] Advocates devote themselves to diagnostic issues, including the inaccuracy of claims that autistics have poor "empathizing" skills (in response to Baron-Cohen 2003), and satirical commentaries on the privileging of "neurotypical" traits in the DSM-IV diagnostic checklist, including the "marked delusional sense of awareness of the existence or feelings of others" (ISNT 1998). They also address more specific questions of rights in employment, treatment, and services.

In 2005, when the Autism Society of America, which calls itself "The Voice of Autism," launched a new campaign for early diagnosis and treatment along with a website, "Getting the Word Out," self-advocates with autism responded indignantly.[8] The website autistics.org changed its slogan to "The Real Voice of Autism," arguing that people with autism ought to speak for themselves and that a diagnosis, rather than familial connections, was the more significant requirement for spokespersons.[9] Parents of children with autism and self-advocates battle over who gets to "speak for" autism, and most importantly, what that speech entails regarding the value of autistic persons and the meaning of their symptoms. While at least one "experimental Aspie school" has been founded where the "aim is to teach students that it is O.K. to 'act autistic' and also how to get by in a world where it is not" (Harmon 2004b), on the other side of the Atlantic, a BBC special on autism that was aired during the summer of 2005 was entitled "Make Me Normal," and featured a school where students were told that their autism was the source of many of the difficulties that they faced in their daily lives. Some of this variance is indeed cultural and national, accounted for by different disciplinary histories of autism research and advocacy, but much of the range of responses is due to the working out of the implications of biosociality around a disorder that is etiologically and phenotypically diverse, imperfectly genetic, and where the symptoms themselves are so socially resonant as to defy easy definition as pathological or merely different. Lenny Schafer, the editor of the Schafer Autism Report and the parent of a child with autism, takes a dim view of self-advocates who disparage "curebies," or parents who seek to treat and cure autism: "I believe, as do others, that it is their autistic-like deficits, the lack of the ability to empathize, that prevents them from seeing what's truly in the hearts of most cure and treatment-loving parents. With love in your heart, you can make mistakes, but you can do little wrong" (Schafer 2005).

Consider, in contrast, the work of Canadian self-advocate Michelle Dawson, who successfully argued in court *against* government funding for behavior modification programs and expressed dismay with the process of diagnosis itself, suggesting that studies of autism prevalence are the proper province of demographers, not epidemiologists, since epidemiology already implies the existence of pathology rather than benign variation (Dawson 2004). Dawson's arguments, like those of ANI, are built on the premise of kinship based on genetic and physiological similarity. She claims kinship with "low-functioning" autistics, arguing that the distinction between low and high-functioning autism is artificial, and that claims about autism as a tragedy serve only to legitimate the failure of organizations devoted to autism to include autistic people in their leadership

(Dawson 2004). Jim Sinclair's essay "Don't Mourn For Us" (1993) continues to express the sentiments of the self-advocacy community, when he writes that parents grieve "the loss of the normal child the parents had hoped and expected to have," but that focus on this grief is damaging:

> Push for the things your expectations tell you are normal, and you'll find frustration, disappointment, resentment, maybe even rage and hatred. Approach respectfully, without preconceptions, and with openness to learning new things, and you will find a world you could never have imagined.
>
> (Sinclair 1993)

Meanwhile, adults with autism have autistic children themselves and reflect on the connections that they have with their children as a result of a shared cognitive world. This is "something fundamental" that they can offer their children as parents and advocates: "[t]hat something is the capability – and importance – of pointing out meaning in autistic behavior, sensory and aesthetic sensibilities, cognitive patterns, and emotional processing – and of asserting their legitimacy" (Schwartz 2004).

Majia Nadesan, the mother of a boy with autism and a thoughtful analyst of these often-conflicting discourses, sees them as representing points of resistance and new possibilities for existence in the twenty-first century (Nadesan 2005). There are few possible responses to autism that do not entail some form of intervention, some set of practices oriented toward the biological entity of autism and an implicit goal of remediation, habilitation, or cure. And even then people with autism may choose unexpectedly when offered the chance to live differently. In Elizabeth Moon's (2003) fantasy novel, *The Speed of Dark*, corporations offer autism-friendly environments complete with trampolines and pinwheels for the comfort of their preternaturally skilled but deeply autistic pattern-recognition specialists. The autistic protagonist, faced with an experimental procedure that might cure him, spends a day in the park paying respectful attention to his heightened, but autistic, sensory perceptions, then decides to undergo the medical procedure and become an astronaut.

Interests, affinities, and the construction of community

Rabinow's concept of biosociality has done much to guide research on the social consequences of new biological knowledge and the "emergent forms of life" (Fischer 1999) that are produced as we come to understand ourselves in terms of our genetic and biological constitutions. The call for empirical research to explore these outcomes is wise. As social scientists, we are as susceptible as genetics researchers and parent organizations to the commercial hype of genomics and the rhetoric of genetic reductionism. The pragmatism of parent organizations should be matched by at least some pragmatism on the part of social scientists, so that we are not caught off guard when the CEO and Executive Director of CAN joins the board of the Autism Treatment Network, making the decision to diversify into treatment research based on identifiable medical problems associated with autism, rather than research on genetics and other "underlying biological mechanisms" (ATN 2004). The public practices of genetics are changing to match the complex findings of genetics research, where genes are merely one link in a cascade between heredity and human experience.

The space between self-advocates and the parent architects of the Autism Genome Project is ultimately an ethical terrain, one that begs exploration by scholars in science studies. Ideals of neurological *diversity* and acceptance do not mesh well with research programs devoted to the eventual treatment or eradication of neurological *disability*, especially in the context of genetics programs that operate according to a relatively impoverished model of genetic causation. While models exist that allow for the modulation of multiple genetic variants by environmental factors, such a model as a basis for community has yet to be fully embraced. Such a representation might lead to the construction of communities around human neurological variation while advocating for the modulation of severe symptoms through a nuanced understanding of developmental environmental genomics. It would take seriously the suffering of those self-advocates who note that far from having a benign condition, they experience severe immune sensitivities, gastrointestinal problems, and other medical conditions possibly associated with their autism, not to mention, among some, the enduring loneliness that comes not from a disinterest in social relations but from a lack of resources for learning where and how to seek them out.

Hannah Landecker argues that exploring the implications of re-engineered and altered life is an important job for historians and anthropologists of biomedicine. She writes that we must ask "[w]hat is the social and cultural task of being biological entities – of being simultaneously biological things and human persons – when 'the biological' is fundamentally plastic?" (Landecker 2006). This plasticity is nowhere more evident than in disorders diagnosed in childhood, where early intervention has the possibility to literally reshape the neurology and biology of the syndrome. The ethical consequences of this plasticity are evident in the fact that whether autism is construed as genetic, psychological, or neurological has consequences for the forms of life that people with autism have access to. Advocates point out that choices to treat children, and what treatments are chosen, literally determine what types of biological persons and adult citizens those children can become. The possibility of intervention is shaped by choices in the framing of autism and the classification of persons with autism. The ethics of interventions are determined by who counts as legitimate spokespersons as a consequence of that framing. As both promoters and critics of the life sciences industry have noted, processes of intervention are always complicated by the unruly tendencies of life forms to evolve beyond their original parameters, making designed forms of life behave in unpredictable ways (Pollack 2006). The recent increase in rates of autism diagnoses may be an instance of "making up people" to fit a quintessentially modern form of pathology, or it may be the unintended consequence of toxic exposures, making people and altering persons in an entirely different sense. Both require that we consider the reality that new forms of life may emerge even when they are unplanned and far from engineered. This realization could constitute the kind of hopeful self-authorship envisioned in some versions of biosociality.

Acknowledgments

I am grateful to Sahra Gibbon, Carlos Novas, and members of the 2005–6 Mellon Foundation seminar on culture and value at Cornell University for their thoughtful comments on drafts of this paper. As always, Susan Lindee and Martha Herbert's advice was invaluable.

Notes

1 By 2005, CAN had contributed over $25 million to research, while NAAR noted that the $21.1 million that it committed in funding "has been leveraged into more than $48 million in autism research awards by the National Institutes of Health (NIH) and other funding sources," NAAR, Available HTTP: http://www.naar.org/research/spons_research.asp (accessed 5 August 2005), and CAN, Available HTTP: http://www.cureautismnow.org/about/index.jsp (accessed 5 August 2005).

2 NAAR uses a two-tiered review process for proposals, with a first review carried out by a board of advisors, after which a "lay review committee" consisting of members of the board of trustees who are family members of people with autism reviews the proposals. CAN maintains similar provisions for input, although the members of their Scientific Review Council must *both* have scientific degrees and be parents of people with autism. Alycia Halladay, Associate Director of research and programs at NAAR, personal communication on 27 December 2005, and Therese Finazzo, Grants Officer, Cure Autism Now, personal communication on 6 January 2006.

3 Linkage studies are generally performed on multiplex families because of the greater likelihood of finding a shared genetic cause for a given disorder in families with multiple cases. My information also comes from a visit to CAN/AGRE headquarters in August 2003, and an interview with Portia Iverson in November 2002.

4 These include the Centers for Professional Excellence in Autism (CPEA), IMGSAC (the International Molecular Genetic Study of Autism Consortium), the Autism Genetics Cooperative (AGC), the Collaborative Programs of Excellence in Autism Research (CPEA), and AGRE.

5 Likewise, Bruno Bettelheim, who had trained in Vienna, was aware of Asperger's work (personal communication, Jacquelyn Sanders, 27 November 2005).

6 www.neurodiversity.com (accessed 26 December 2005), www.autistics.org (accessed 26 December 2005), and http://www.aspiesforfreedom.com (accessed 26 December 2005), as well as http://undergroundaspergian.tripod.com/passing/ (accessed 26 December 2005).

7 http://www.autistart.com/designlist.htm (accessed 26 December 2005). For the "autism awareness" ribbon, see www.autism-society.org (accessed 26 December 2005).

8 http://www.autism-society.org/site/PageServer (accessed 26 December 2005), and http://www.gettingthewordout.org/home.php (accessed 26 December 2005).

9 http://www.autistics.org/ (accessed 26 December 2005).

Bibliography

AGRE (undated) Available HTTP: http://www.agre.org (accessed 3 July 2003).

American Psychiatric Association (2000) *Diagnostic and Statistical Manual of Mental Disorders: DSM-IV-TR* (fourth edition, text revision). Washington, DC: American Psychiatric Association.

Asperger, H. ([1944] 1991) "'Autistic Psychopathy' in Childhood," Uta Frith (ed.) *Autism and Asperger Syndrome*. Cambridge: Cambridge University Press: 88.

Autism Society of America (2005) "Getting the Word Out." Available HTTP: http://www.gettingthewordout.org (accessed 4 July 2006).

Autism Treatment Network (2004) Available HTTP: http://www.autismtreatmentnetwork.org/about.htm#Why%20ATN%20Is%20Needed%20Now (accessed 28 January 2006).

Baron-Cohen, S. (2003) *The Essential Difference: the Truth About the Male and Female Brain*. New York: Perseus Books Group.

Bettelheim, B. (1967) *The Empty Fortress: Infantile Autism and the Birth of the Self.* New York: The Free Press.

Callon, M. (1987) "Some Elements of a Sociology of Translation: Domestication of the Scallops and the Fishermen of St. Brieuc Bay," in J. Law (ed.) *Power, Action and Belief: A New Sociology of Knowledge*. London: Routledge and Kegan Paul.

CAN press release. Available HTTP: http://www.cureautismnow.org/site/apps/nl/content2.asp?c=bhLOK2PILuF&b=1289185&ct=2676321&tr=y&auid=1771171 (accessed 11 July 2006).

CAN fundraising pamphlet (2003) "Cure Autism Now," 5455 Wilshire Blvd, Los Angeles, CA.

CAN press release (2007) "Autism Speaks and Cure Autism Now Complete Merger: Combined Operations of Leading Autism Organizations Will Lead to Enhanced Research, Treatment and Advocacy Programs." Available HTTP: http://www.cureautismnow.org/site/apps/nl/content2.asp?c=bhLOK2PILuF&b=1841353&ct=3523475 (accessed 19 March 2007).

CAN website. Available HTTP: http://www.cureautismnow.org/about/index.jsp (accessed 5 August 2005).

Dawson, G., Webb, S., Schellenberg, G.D., Dager, S., Friedman, S., Aylward, E., Richards, T. (2002) "Defining the Broader Phenotype of Autism: Genetic, Brain, and Behavioral Perspectives," *Development and Psychopathology*, 14: 581–611.

Dawson, M. (2004) "Being Told or Being Told Off? Reciprocity at the Diagnostic Interview." Available HTTP: http://www.sentex.net/~nexus23/naa_bto.html (accessed 31 January 2006).

Dawson, M., Mottron, L., Jelenic, P. and Soulières, I. (2005) "Superior Performance of Autistics on RPM and PPVT Relative to Wechsler Scales Provides Evidence for the Nature of Autistic Intelligence." Poster presented at the International Meeting for Autism Research, Boston, MA. Available HTTP: http://www.sentex.net/~nexus23/naa_imfar.html (accessed 3 July 2006).

Dekker. M. (1999) "On Our Own Terms: Emerging Autistic Culture." Available HTTP: http://trainland.tripod.com/martijn.htm (accessed 14 October 2004).

Epstein, S. (1995) "The Construction of Lay Expertise: AIDS Activism and the Forging of Credibility in the Reform of Clinical Trials," *Science, Technology, and Human Values*, 20(4), Special Issue: Constructivist Perspectives on Medical Work: Medical Practices and Science and Technology Studies: 408–37.

Fischer, M.M.J. (1999) "Emergent Forms of Life: Anthropologies of Late or Post-Modernities," *Annual Review of Anthropology*, 28: 455–78.

Fombonne, E. (2001) "Is There an Epidemic of Autism?" *Pediatrics*, 107: 411–12.

Frith, U. (1989) *Autism: Explaining the Enigma*. Oxford: Basil Blackwell.

Frith, U. (1991) "Asperger and His Syndrome," in U. Frith (ed.) *Autism and Asperger Syndrome*. Cambridge: Cambridge University Press.

Gernsbacher, M.A., Dawson, M. and Goldsmith, H.H. (2005) "Three reasons not to believe in an autism epidemic," *Current Directions in Pyschological Science*, 14(2): 55–8.

Geschwind, D.H., Sowinski, J., Lord, C., Iversen, P., Shestack, J., Jones, P., Ducat, L. and Spence, S.J. (2001) AGRE Steering Committee. "The Autism Genetic Resource Exchange: A Resource for the Study of Autism and Related Neuropsychiatric Conditions," *American Journal of Human Genetics*, 69(2): 463–6.

Grandin, T. (2004). *Developing Talents: Careers for Individuals with Asperger Syndrome and High-Functioning Autism.* Shawnee Mission, KS: Autism Asperger Publishing Company.

Hacking, I. (1999) "Making Up People," in M. Biagioli (ed.) *The Science Studies Reader*. New York: Routledge.

Hacking, I . (2000). *The Social Construction of What?* Cambridge, MA: Harvard University Press.

Hacking, I. (2006) "What is Tom Saying to Maureen?" *London Review of Books*, 28(9). Available HTTP: http://www.lrb.co.uk/v28/n09/hack01_.html (accessed 3 July 2006).

Harmon, A. (2004a) "Finding Out: Adults and Autism; An Answer, But Not a Cure, For A Social Disorder," *The New York Times*, 29 April.

Harmon, A. (2004b) "How About Not 'Curing' Us, Some Autistics Are Pleading," *The New York Times*, 20 December.

Hedgecoe, A. (2001) "Schizophrenia and the Narrative of Enlightened Geneticization," *Social Studies of Science*, 31(6): 875–911.

Institute for the Study of the Neurologically Typical (ISNT) (1998) "666.00 Neurotypic Disorder." Available HTTP: http://isnt.autistics.org/dsn.html (accessed 26 December 2005).

Inose, K. and Fukushima, M. (2005) "Asperger's Solitary Ally: Psychiatric Debate and the Educational Policy on Autism in Postwar Japan." Presentation at the Society for the Social Studies of Science (4S), Fall 2005.

Kanner, L. (1943) "Autistic Disturbances of Affective Contact," *Nervous Child*, 2: 217–50.

Kirby, D. (2005) *Evidence of Harm. Mercury in Vaccines and the Autism Epidemic: A Medical Controversy*. New York: St Martin's Press.

Landecker, H. (2006) "Living Differently in Time: Plasticity, Temporality and Cellular Bioetchnologies," *Culture Machine: Generating Research in Culture and Theory*. Available HTTP: http://culturemachine.tees.ac.uk/Cmach/Backissues/j007/Articles/landecker.htm (accessed 3 July 2006).

Merton, R.K. (1942) "The Normative Structure of Science," in N.W. Storer (ed.) *The Sociology of Science* (1973) Chicago, IL: University of Chicago Press: 267–78.

Moon, E. (2003) *The Speed of Dark*. New York: Ballantine Books.

Mulkay, M. (1976) "Norms and ideology of science," *Social Science Information*, 15(4–5): 637–56.

Nadesan, M. (2005) *Constructing Autism: Unraveling the "Truth" and Understanding the Social*. New York: Routledge.

National Alliance for Autism Research (NAAR) (2004) "NAAR Autism Genome Project: Frequently Asked Questions." Available HTTP: http://www.naar.org/news/render_pr.asp?intNewsItemID=176 (accessed 3 July 2006).

National Alliance for Autism Research (NAAR) (2005a) "Autism Speaks and the National Alliance for Autism Research (NAAR) Complete Merger." Available HTTP: http://www.naar.org/news/render_pr.asp?intNewsItemID=335 (accessed 4 July 2006).

National Alliance for Autism Research (NAAR) (2005b) "NAAR Sponsored Research." Available HTTP: http://www.naar.org/research/spons_research_2004.htm (accessed 4 July 2006).

National Alliance for Autism Research (NAAR) (undated) "NAAR Autism Genome Project: Fact Sheet." National Alliance for Autism Research. Available HTTP: http://www.naar.org/news/render_pr.asp?intNewsItemID=176 (accessed 3 July 2006).

National Alliance for Autism Research (NAAR) website. Available HTTP: <http://www.naar.org/research/spons_research.asp> (accessed 5 August 2005).

Park, C. (1967) *The Siege: A Family's Journey Into the World of An Autistic Child*. Boston, MA: Little, Brown, and Co.

Pollack, A. (2006) "Custom-Made Microbes, at Your Service," *The New York Times*, 17 January.

Rabinow, P. (1996a) *Making PCR: A Story of Biotechnology*. Chicago, IL and London: University of Chicago Press.

Rabinow. P. (1996b) "Artificiality and Enlightenment: from Sociobiology to Biosociality," in *Essays on the Anthropology of Reason.* Princeton, NJ: Princeton University Press.

Rapp, R. (1999) *Testing Women, Testing the Fetus: The Social Impact of Amniocentesis in America*. New York: Routledge.

Rapp, R. (2000) "Extra chromosomes and blue tulips: medico-familial interpretations," in M. Lock, A. Young and A. Cambrosio (eds) *Living and Working with the New Medical Technologies: Intersections of Inquiry*. Cambridge: Cambridge University Press: 184–207.

Rapp, R. and Ginsburg, F. (2001) "Enabling Disability: Rewriting Kinship, Reimagining Citizenship," *Public Culture*, 13(3): 533–56.

Rose, N. and Novas, C. (2003) "Biological Citizenship," in A. Ong and S. Collier (eds) *Global Anthropology*. Oxford: Blackwell. Available HTTP: http://www.lse.ac.uk/collections/sociology/pdf/RoseandNovasBiologicalCitizenship2002.pdf (accessed 3 July 2006).

Schafer, L. (2005) "Response to Letters: Somewhere over the Spectrum, Part 3," *Schafer Autism Report* (11 January 2005). Available HTTP: http://lists.envirolink.org/pipermail/sareport/Week-of-Mon-20050110/000350.html (accessed 26 December 2005).

Schwartz, P. (2004) "Wearing Two Hats: On Being a Parent and On the Spectrum Myself." The article first appeared in the MAAP newsletter, 2004, Volume ii (www.maapservices.org). Available HTTP: http://www.autistics.org/cap/twohats.html (accessed 26 December 2005).

Schwartz, P. (2006) "Working Models for Developing an Ally Network: Outreach and Support for Straight Allies in the Gay Community." Presentation at Autreat 2006, Philadelphia, PA.

Silverman, C. and Herbert, M. (2003) "Autism and Genetics," *GeneWatch*, 16(1). Available HTTP: http://www.gene-watch.org/genewatch/articles/16-2herbert_silverman.html.

Sinclair, J. (1993) "Don't Mourn For Us," originally published in the Autism Network International newsletter, *Our Voice*, 1(3). Available HTTP: http://ani.autistics.org/dont_mourn.html (26 December 2005).

Sinclair, J. (2005) "Autism Network International: the Development of a Community and its Culture." Available HTTP: http://web.syr.edu/~jisincla/History_of_ANI.html (accessed 8 December 2005).

Smith, Jonathan, dir. (2004) Documentary Film: "Only Human: Make Me Normal," Century Films for Channel 4 (aired 2 June 2004).

Stacey, P. (2003) *The Boy Who Loved Windows: Opening the Heart and Mind of a Child Threatened with Autism*. Cambridge, MA: Da Capo Press.

Veenstra-VanderWeele, J. and Cook, E.H. (2004) "Review: Molecular Genetics of Autism Spectrum Disorder," *Mol Psychiatry*, 9(9): 819–32.

Wieder, S. and Greenspan, S.I. (2003) "Climbing the symbolic ladder in the DIR model through floor time/interactive play," *Autism*, 7(4): 425–35.

Wing, L. (1981) "Asperger's Syndrome: A Clinical Account," *Psychological Medicine*, 11: 115–29.

Zitner, A. (2003) "Whose DNA Is It, Anyway?" *LA Times*, 18 July.

3 Biosociality and susceptibility genes

A cautionary tale

Margaret Lock

> I ... now see my reluctance to apply the term Alzheimer's to my father as a way of protecting the specificity of Earl Franzen from the generality of a named condition. Conditions have symptoms; symptoms point to the organic basis of everything we are. They point to the brain as meat. And, where I ought to recognize that, yes, the brain is meat, I seem instead to maintain a blind spot across which I then interpolate stories that emphasize the more soul-like aspects of the self.
>
> Jonathan Franzen, "My Father's Brain," *The New Yorker*,
> 10 September 2001: 85

In 1906 when Alois Alzheimer first presented the case history of 51-year-old Augusta Deter, his conclusion was that her condition was an anomaly – simply an unusual example of the then well recognized disease of senile dementia that had manifested itself at a remarkably early age. Initially, Alzheimer did not apparently believe that he had come across a "new" disease. It was Emil Kraepelin who, in the 1910 edition of his influential textbook on psychiatry, was the first to make a cautious, but nevertheless clear distinction between presenile and senile dementia, naming the former condition as Alzheimer's disease. At the time, Alzheimer was working as part of Kraepelin's group, and it is unclear to this day as to whether Alzheimer and Kraepelin were by this time of a like mind or not. Moreover, arguments persist among historians as to exactly why Kraepelin decided to lay claim to the discovery of a new disease; some insist that it was primarily to enhance the reputation of his group and the use of their particular scientific methods, but others believe that the story is more complex, and that much remains unknown (Ballenger 2006; Beach1987; Holstein 1997).

Between the 1960s and 1980s four innovative changes took place contributing to the eventual establishment of a broad based consensus among scientists that Alzheimer's is a bona fide, distinct disease and, moreover, not only presenile dementia, but the much more common senile dementia be labeled as such. Even so, arguments persist to the present day as to whether Alzheimer's is, in the end, merely a phenomenon of aging – simply the signs of senility evident in us all if we live long enough (Breitner 1999; Whitehouse 2001). And, further, if Alzheimer's is indeed a disease, then what exactly *are* its distinctive pathological features? Many other conditions exhibit the distinctive neurofibillary plaques and tangles associated with Alzheimer's disease, including Parkinson's disease, Down syndrome, various toxic conditions, and so on. Adding to the confusion, autopsies of the brains of deceased non-demented people regularly exhibit these same plaques and tangles (Ince 2001).

Despite these well recognized medical discrepancies, a combination of technological advancements and social and political pressures brought about the consolidation of a dominant position in the second half of the twentieth century, namely that Alzheimer's disease is not only uncontrovertibly real, but a disease to be feared, particularly given the aging of so many populations (Ballenger 2006). The first significant change was the development of the electron microscope, permitting refinements in classification of neuropathologies. Second, in the 1970s, the influential neurologist, Robert Katzman, publicly insisted that received wisdom of the time be abandoned, namely that growing old inevitably results in dementia. Katzman also declared that *all* cases of senility should be recognized as pathology, labeled as Alzheimer's disease, and understood as entirely distinct from normal aging (1976). Third, was the formation in the United States of the National Institute of Aging (NIA), founded specifically to foster a comprehensive research program on ageing. Fourth, was the emergence of an incipient Alzheimer's movement, and its consolidation commencing from 1977 as the Alzheimer's disease and Related Disorders Association (ADRDA), with the strong support of the first director of the NIA, the gerontologist and psychiatrist, Robert Butler. The activities of the ADRDA in turn increased the legitimacy of the NIA in large part because it lobbied government and actively set about raising money for research into Alzheimer's disease (Fox 1989).

The sociologist Patrick Fox points out that interest in the newly formed organization began to explode in 1980 after a letter from a family member of an Alzheimer's disease patient was published in the nationally syndicated column *Dear Abby.* Following this publication, the ADRDA received more than 30,000 letters, precipitating interest among the public in this new disease as nothing else before it had done (Fox 1989). Jonathan Franzen notes in the New Yorker article cited above that when the term "Alzheimer's disease" was first achieving currency he was concerned about yet further "medicalization of human experience, the latest entry in the ever-expanding nomenclature of victimhood" (2001: 85). Franzen admits that, fifteen years later, he still feels uneasy, even though he recognizes that it is comforting to know that millions of other people's parents suffer from this appalling condition, making them at times an embarrassment to their children. But having a parent who is demented, above all, will always be a very personal exierience, declares Franzen, and for this reason any comfort obtained from simply naming the condition is limited, especially because, in the case of Alzheimer's disease, a diagnosis does not result in effective treatment.

This observation by Franzen is of significance when considering the concept of biosociality, especially the way in which it has been played out with respect to Alzheimer's disease. Once the disease was "discovered," medicalized, and the ADRDA founded, a pattern of biosociality was soon established that remains in place today. The international Alzheimer Association and its national and regional subsidiaries continue the work of lobbying, raising funds, and promoting research and public education that was started in the 1970s. Regional chapters hold workshops, offer courses, and organize public lectures, and many are also involved with educational programs designed for health professionals, including primary care physicians. But the principal work of these chapters is the generation of support networks for affected families. However, due in large part to the late age of onset of most cases of AD, and the characteristic symptomatology of memory loss and disorientation that becomes progressively more debilitating, ending in death, it is not usually patients who come together in support groups (as might be the case, for example, with breast cancer or HIV), with the exception only of those people in the very early stages of Alzheimer's. Groups are designed principally to give support and advice to families and caregivers of patients (Gubrium 2000). It is in these weekly meetings that a form of biosociality takes place among families affected by this disease, but discussion is primarily about how to take the car keys away from a stricken relative without destroying their dignity, abuse by demented parents of middle aged children acting as care-givers, incontinence, and other behavioral matters. The possible cause or causes of Alzheimer's disease, including discussion about whether or not genes are implicated, do not occupy a great deal of time in support groups. Care giving, the search for medication, and discussion of possible measures to slow down disease progression are of prime concern.

Pamphlets from AD societies in the United States, Canada, and the United Kingdom all relegate the topic of genetics to a brief paragraph or two, often at the end of their documents, and testing for the one gene consistently associated with late onset Alzheimer's disease is actively discouraged (Alzheimer's Association 2002; Alzheimer Society of Canada 2002; Alzheimer Society 2003, 2005 http://www.alzheimers.org.uk). Above all, it is the experience of caring for someone who is demented, learning about the latest medications, coping with the crises of daily life, and eventual placement in a nursing home that draws involved families to an AD society. But it is noteworthy that, despite the presence of branches of the AD Society in virtually every city and even in many large towns in North America, by far the majority of families affected by Alzheimer's disease choose *not* to participate in support groups. The reason in many cases is that people are simply too busy; or because they rely entirely on family networks for support, supplemented by information gleaned from acquaintances, neighbors, the internet or elsewhere; alternatively, outright denial is often evident in the early stages of the disease (Novek unpublished thesis), or shame and stigma are associated with having a demented family member. Another reason given by several people when interviewed is that they do not want to sit around in a group and listen to other people's troubles and/or they dislike participating in an activity that seems to them to be the equivalent of psychological counseling (Lock *et al.* in press).

Probably the main reason why AD societies play down discussion about the genetics of Alzheimers and, in particular, consideration of genetic testing, is because their administrators are following official guidelines. These guidelines, put out by medical organizations, and also by the national AD societies of the United

States, Canada, the United Kingdom, and France, state that genetic testing for late onset AD should not be routinely performed (Agence Nationale d'Accréditation et d'Évaluation en Santé (ANAES) 2000; Health Canada; 2001; *Journal of the American Medical Association* 1995; McConnell *et al.* 1998; Relkin *et al.* 1996). Such recommendations are easily justified because there is no known prevention or treatment for AD that is more than minimally effective, and learning the genetic status of a patient has no effect on clinical care, although occasionally the test is carried out to add support to a problematic diagnosis.

The result is that, although many people now firmly believe that genetics are involved in Alzheimer's disease (although most do not believe that genetics *determine* the disease (Lock *et al.* 2005)), family members are not encouraged to discuss concerns about their own "embodied risk" more than minimally in AD society support groups. Moreover, if and when individuals raise questions about the genetics of AD with their family doctors, they are usually strongly discouraged from seeking out testing because this practice is not recommended by the medical establishment. Testing for late onset Alzheimer's disease is not covered by government funded health care systems, and can only be accomplished by seeking out a company advertising the service online for a cost of several thousand dollars. This type of genetic testing is usually offered with no follow-up advice or counseling. The combination of AD society activities functioning primarily in order to assist with care giving and strong discouragement of genetic testing by both the AD societies and the medical establishment means that a form of biosociality based on shared DNA characteristics is effectively blocked for relatives of individuals affected by Alzheimer's disease. And, I would argue, for reasons that will become apparent below, if and when testing slowly becomes routinized, biosociality based on DNA typing is still unlikely to take place. Moreover, the persistence among many families of stigma and shame in connection with this disease, coupled with a strong disinclination on the part of many people to participate in activities that they characterize as psychological counseling, effectively blocks *any* form of biosociality beyond the immediate family for the majority of people dealing with Alzheimer's disease.

Genetic hype and hope

In a 1997 article entitled "Plundered Memories," published in the now defunct journal *The Sciences*, Zaven Khachaturian, the Director of the Ronald and Nancy Reagan Research Institute of the Alzheimer's Association had this to say:

> Some critics ask whether genetic research is worth the resources it consumes and the anguish it will bring to those who test positive for a harmful gene – when a cure still seems so far away. In my view, however, the genetic approach is on the right track, and I think the continuing research on Alzheimer's disease may soon confirm that belief. Those of us in the front lines of the fight against Alzheimer's have never been closer to unmasking this mysterious thief, the robber of the very thing that makes human beings unique.
>
> (Khachaturian 1997: 21)

In the same year, 1997, John Hardy, who researches the genetics of Alzheimer's disease, and is currently chief of the laboratory of Neurogenetics at the National Institute of Aging argued, "we now know several *causes* (emphasis added) of Alzheimer's disease (all of them genetic)." Hardy had in mind both early onset Alzheimer's disease, in which genes with an autosomally dominant mode of transmission are invariably involved, *and* late onset Alzheimer's disease in which the implicated susceptibility gene is involved in approximately somewhere between 30 percent and 60 percent of all instances of the disease. In 1997 Hardy could not be faulted for under-estimating the complexity of action of this latter gene, and he apparently had no compunction about stating, "… the unofficial "goal" of the NIA is to have some form of effective therapy by the year 2000 and this goal may yet be realized" (1997). Hardy assumed that the recent genetic insights of the time would bring about a therapeutic breakthrough but, as is well known, effective medication for AD has yet to be found, even though research into the genetics of dementia has accelerated exponentially since the end of the twentieth century.

The genetics of Alzheimer's disease

Alois Alzheimer originally observed a case of what is now known as "early onset" Alzheimer's disease. This form of dementia occurs in only about 170 extended families world wide, has long been thought of as a "genetic disease," and is associated with three specific, genetic mutations that have all been mapped (St George-Hyslop 2000). It is not strictly true to claim that the gene determines even this autosomal dominant form of the disease, because the age of onset for identical twins can vary by as much as a decade (Tilley *et al.* 1998). Early onset AD usually (but not inevitably) manifests itself somewhere between the ages of 35 and 60, progresses relatively quickly to death, and accounts for between 2 and 5 percent of all diagnosed cases of the disease.

In 1993 the first publication appeared that explicitly made an association between the APOE gene and an increased risk for the common, late onset form of AD (Corder *et al.* 1993). This finding forced some revisions of the received wisdom of the time – namely that Alzheimer's disease in older people is "sporadic," and does not "run in families." The APOE gene, present in all mammals, is located in humans on chromosome 19, and is essential for lipid metabolism. This gene comes in three forms APOEε2, APOEε3, and APOEε4 that are universally distributed, and evidence from over 100 laboratories indicates that it is the APOEε4 allele that puts one at increased risk for AD. Between 14 and 16 percent of Caucasian populations (the most extensively studied biological population) carry at least one ε4 allele, however, it is unanimously agreed that the presence of the allele is neither necessary nor sufficient to cause the disease, for reasons that are as yet very poorly understood. It is estimated that at least 50 percent of ε4 carriers never get Alzheimer's disease. Research in connection with the allele shows that when it *is* implicated in AD, exactly the same final biological pathway is involved as that set in motion by the autosomal dominant genes associated with the early onset form of the disease; but the biological changes in which APOEε4 in its homozygous form is implicated become manifest later in life, usually between the ages of 65 and 75 (Selkoe 2002). For individuals who are heterozygous and have only one ε4 allele, the age of onset is later. Given that somewhere between 30 and 60 percent of patients diagnosed with late onset AD do not have the APOEε4 allele (Myers *et al.* 1996), there must be at least one other, and probably several more pathways to Alzheimer's disease. It is assumed that such pathways are constituted by mutually interactive genes and non-coding DNA, in conjunction with environmental factors, internal and/or external to the body. These alternative pathways become evident late in life, usually after age 70 or later, but they too result in the same final common pathway as that for early onset and APOEε4 linked AD, with the characteristic pathological signs that can only be seen at autopsy – plaques, tangles, and cell loss in the brain. Because, in addition to APOEε4, it is assumed that several more genes must be implicated in late onset AD, intensive gene hunting continues unabated.

The current situation has recently been summarized by two neurogeneticists as follows: "First, and most importantly, the heritability of AD is high … this has been demonstrated in various studies … over the past decades." But, these experts go on to note, "most of the research currently being done has faulty methodology, lacks replication, and is inattentive to haplotype structure" (Bertram and Tanzi 2004: R135). Using the citation index PubMed, Bertram and Tanzi show that in 2003 alone a total of 1,037 studies were carried out on the genetics of AD, out of which 55 analyzed genes were reported to have a positive association with increased risk for the disease, while 68 tested negative. Candidate genes have been examined on every single chromosome and mitochondrial DNA has also been investigated. These authors conclude with a caveat: "while the genetic association *per se* [of APOEε4 with AD] has been extremely well established … there is no consensus as to *how* this association translates pathophysiologically," nor how it functions in conjunction with the other numerous candidate genes (Bertram and Tanzi 2004: R137).

Until recently, because the disease is limited to older people, and because researchers thought that it was sporadic in origin, few pedigree studies with large extended families have been carried out in connection with late onset AD. Now that the results of such research are beginning to accrue, the inconclusive nature of knowledge about APOE is glaringly evident. In an isolated Dutch family, for example, where numerous cases of five different kinds of dementia have been diagnosed, the APOEε4 allele is present in the family with greater frequency than usual, but only 45 percent of the identified cases of late onset AD are carriers of this allele (Sleegers *et al.* 2004). The more such articles are published, a clear impression is created that too much weight may have been given by researchers to the contribution of the APOEε4 allele to AD, although at the same time research continues to show that this allele is indeed regularly implicated in both familial and sporadic forms of AD, and also in heart disease. The biological anthropologist, Alan Templeton, is particularly critical of the conclusions drawn by most researchers in connection with APOE function. He points out that genomes are "commonly organized into clusters of functionally related genes" and that APOE is part of one such cluster. Templeton argues that when this type of gene is associated by linkage with a specific phenotype great caution is called for, because the gene may simply be a marker for another gene or genes located nearby on the same, clustered segment of DNA (Templeton 1998: 376).

Even given the obvious complexity, the genetic epidemiologist, Richard Mayeux commenting on the genetics of AD in a recent New Yorker article, made it clear that he does not believe we will be held back too much longer from more insightful knowledge: "a decade from now your doctor will look up your gene profile and decide whether you have a high risk for Alzheimer's, and then give you a prophylactic treatment of some sort." He adds, "Right now, you don't know what the hell to do!" (Halpern 2005).

Despite this optimism, population research in connection with the genetics of both early and late onset AD suggests that no straightforward solution is in sight; this epidemiologically-based approach to the problem has amply demonstrated that genes are shape-shifters without peer, the products of evolutionary and recent human history, dietary and climatic patterns, possibly of toxic environments and, at times, of serendipitous mutations. Most epidemiological research into the genetics of AD has been carried out since the early 1990s, when the significance of the ApOEε4 allele was first identified but, as noted above, these studies have been confined largely to so-called Caucasian populations (Growden 1998; Korovaitseva *et al.* 2001; Roses 1998; Saunders 2000; Silverman *et al.* 2003). Even though the methodology has been criticized, this research makes it clear that the relationship between ApOEε4 and AD incidence is probably significantly weaker than commonly suggested. One community-based study found that 85 percent of elderly homozygous ε4 individuals whose average age was 81 showed no sign of dementia when given the standard tests for cognitive functioning (Hyman *et al.* 1996).

Adding to the uncertainties, ApOEε4 has been shown to work in unexpected ways in specific populations. Among Pygmies and other groups of people whose subsistence economy was until relatively recently predominantly that of hunting and gathering, possession of an ApOEε4 genotype *apparently* protects against AD. This finding holds when controlled for age (Corbo and Scacchi 1999). Low rates of AD have been reported for parts of Nigeria, and the presence of an ε4 allele does not appear to place individuals at increased risk (Farrer *et al.* 1997). On the other hand, ApOEε4 is significantly associated with dementia among African Americans, although less so than in Caucasian populations (Farrer 2000). Once again, the methodology of this research has been criticized, but the data appear sufficiently robust to conclude that risk reducing factors (in Africa) *and* risk enhancing factors (in North America) must be implicated, among them other genes, their protein products, diet, environment, and quite possibly yet other variables.

It is evident that basic science and epidemiological findings about late onset Alzheimer's disease are subject to continual revision and are far from conclusive. It is no surprise, then, that current guidelines about genetic testing for APOE status do not support its routinization in clinical care, but it is possible that this may change in the not too distant future. Very recently *The Pharmacogenetics Journal* presented preliminary findings concerning a new drug, Rosiglitazone (Risner *et al*. 2006) This drug alters glucose metabolism in the brain and, it is reported, has a positive effect on cognitive functioning, but only on those patients with mild to moderate AD who are APOEɛ3. This finding, by the team of Allan Roses who was the first to report that APOEɛ4 puts individuals at increased risk for AD, and who is now the CEO of the pharmaceutical company GlaxoSmithKline, suggests that, *should* this drug move successfully through clinical trials, AD genotyping will likely become routinized in clinical settings. Other researchers are working on similar drugs believed to function differentially according to genotype.

What does the current state of knowledge about AD genetics imply for the concepts of biosociality and subjectivity, for the present and in the future? Clearly, learning that you carry an APOEɛ4 allele should not precipitate an effect so marked, as surely must be the case on learning that one carries one of the genes associated with early onset Alzheimer's disease, or the toxic form of the gene associated with Huntington's disease. Learning about one's APOE status does not provide information about a highly probable future; it only raises a possible scenario, one that anyone living in a family where AD is present has already entertained at some point in their life.

Embodying a predisposition

Novas and Rose argue that, as a result of recent advances in the life sciences, including human genetics and genetic medicine, a "mutation in personhood" has come about (2000: 485). This transformation is not, they argue, merely a modification of lay, professional, and scientific ideas about human identity and subjectivity, but is also a shift in "presuppositions about human beings that are embedded in and underpin particular practices." One result is the emergent figure of an individual "genetically at risk" (2000: 486).

Ian Hacking's concept of dynamic nominalism permits some further elaboration on what kind of individual this might be. His position is that "a kind of person" comes into being at the same time as the "kind of being itself" is invented; "in some cases ... our classifications and our classes conspire to emerge hand in hand, each egging the other on" (1986: 228). On the basis of an examination of the history of several medical conditions, Hacking concludes that it is by no means the case that people are "made up" as specific groupings and as named types simply because they become classified this way by bureaucrats, medical experts, or other powerful bodies, that they then come to embody. Hacking argues that the social categories we create are not static and, second, and most important, that they do not arise in any straightforward way out of the human mind. Hacking uses the concept of dynamic nominalism to gloss his own position, one in which nature is given its due – in other words, many categories (planets, horses, and so on) "come from nature" although, of course, humans then tinker with taxonomic classifications – the dementias, including Alzheimer's disease, is an excellent example of this process.

With remarkable rapidity, as genomic technologies advance, segments of DNA are being marked out as "natural" signifiers for who among us should be counted as genetically at risk but, we now know, DNA segments are rarely, and possibly never, *determinants* of disease, as was formerly assumed to be the case. Taxonomic classifications of and predictions about future disease based on DNA typing are, for the moment at least, in flux and under revision, with the result that neither the construction of risk estimates about named diseases, nor the actual practices associated with emerging genomic knowledge, are stable or uniform.[1] The APOE gene, although one of the best worked out examples of a susceptibility gene nevertheless is an exemplar of unpredictability; the activities of this segment of DNA make it patently clear that when dealing with the genetics of complex disease, recognition of dynamic nominalism – the co-construction of the material and the social – is indispensable. In other words, estimates about future risk and the effects on an individual of being informed about such risk, together with possible associated transformations in embodied identity and practices of self-governance, cannot be assessed independently of the "non-human actor" (Latour 1993) – the DNA segment – and the environment in which it is functioning.

The hype of future innovations and hope for therapeutic discoveries that accompanied the findings of molecular genetics at the end of the last century has dissolved in the first years of the present century in a wave of uncertainty. Rapidly expanding functional genomics has demonstrated very quickly how misguided was the earlier overly simplistic thinking supported by many scientists (Lock 2005; Moss 2003; Rose 2005). A great deal of fine-tuning is urgently needed if social science commentary about the effects of postgenomic knowledge on human behavior and subjective understanding is to be effective. One way to accomplish this is to focus in detail on specific named conditions (provided that due attention is given to the historical and social construction and labeling of diseases). For example, the age of onset of a condition and its specific pathological effects should be taken into account. People do not respond in the same way to being told that they are at risk for a disease that manifests itself late in life as compared to one that has an impact on reproductive decisions. And being informed about one's genetic heritage while pregnant is entirely different from being told about it in late middle age. Moreover, learning that you have an autosomal dominant gene for a deadly disease that will almost certainly be expressed, is by no means the same kind of knowledge as being told that you have a susceptibility gene that may, under poorly understood circumstances, put you at a life-time increased risk of approximately 30 percent over a "normal" population.

It is well recognized today that genetic testing is not merely an individual matter, but inevitably has broader social consequences, not the least of which being that results have undeniable implications for kin, in addition to which are possible work and insurance related repercussions. Experience of stigma and discrimination in daily life may also be among the negative effects (Duster 1990; Nelkin and Tancredi 1989; Offit *et al.* 2004; Zick *et al.* 2005).

As Paul Rabinow has pointed out, people learn about genetics from a number of sources – the medical world, advocacy groups, the media, direct-to-consumer advertising, from friends, relatives, public forums, and on the street (1994). They usually have time to reflect on what they have heard, are not pressed into taking immediate action and, more often than not, are particularly interested in gleaning information about one or more specific diseases that they believe "run" in their families. Given that basic science findings are very often unstable and inconclusive, people's decisions about testing will be influenced by the way in which and exactly what knowledge is imparted to them. Questions that arise immediately are whether or not families are made aware of the molecular complexity; of the inability, in most cases, of experts to predict either the severity of the disease or, for complex diseases, if the condition will occur at all.

In summary, being told that one is genetically at risk potentially raises a spectrum of concerns and responses that are embedded in and informed by material, medical, familial, social, political, historical and other variables, no doubt at times, some of them serendipitous. These many aspects of the biosocial are in need of empirical investigation. To engage with the effects of genotyping on subjectivity and the social, leaving other broader considerations black boxed, is to risk being drawn uncritically into the hype associated with genes and genomics. On the other hand biosociality writ large, something akin to the idea of "distributed bio-sociality" discussed by Gibbon and Novas in the introduction, is good to think with; I would argue that a concept such as this, in concert with recognition of the co-production of the material and socio/political, is probably indispensable to the social sciences if commentary about genomics is not to be reduced entirely to a rehash of medical hype and hope and related disputes internal to the world of the biosciences. One further cautionary note is in order, hinted at above: investigation in connection with the responses of many people living with a family member diagnosed with Alzheimer's disease shows that the result is, if anything, a reduced sociality. People actively reduce their social networks under pressures of various kinds, among them work demands, care giving, shame, and private resort to the internet for information.[2]

Genetic testing for late onset Alzheimer's disease

Even though official guidelines are currently opposed to routine testing for the APOE gene, several private companies offer testing (the US based Athena diagnostics holds the patent for APOE testing), and an "Early Alert Alzheimer's Home Screening Test" kit is marketed directly to consumers (Kier and Molinari 2003). Furthermore, a strong argument is being made among certain neurologists that individuals diagnosed with Mild Cognitive Impairment (believed to be a sign of incipient Alzhemer's disease) should be routinely tested for their APOE status. Recent research suggests that although by no means everyone diagnosed with MCI "converts" to AD, those diagnosed individuals who also have the ε4 allele are at much greater risk for conversion, and should be identified as early as possible (Farlow *et al.* 2004). In addition to testing carried out in these settings, an NIH approved randomized controlled trial involving APOE testing that goes under the name of REVEAL (Risk Evaluation and Education for Alzheimer's disease) is in progress. Families where one or more members have been diagnosed with Alzheimer's disease are subjects for this research. Data extracted from ethnographic interviews with 65 of these research subjects will be presented as the concluding part of this chapter.

The REVEAL trial was originally a three -sited project involving 162 subjects at Boston University Medical School, Case Western Reserve, Cleveland, and Cornell University Medical School, New York, but has been extended to include Howard University in Washington DC. Subjects for this trial were recruited either through systematic ascertainment from American AD research registries kept at the respective medical schools, or through self-referral at each site (Cupples *et al.* 2004). Upon recruitment into Phase 1 of the project, research subjects were randomized into intervention and control groups. In the original three-sited sample everyone self-identified as "white," and the majority are women. Participants are highly educated, with a mean of 17 years of education. The Howard sample identify themselves as African Americans, and also have a high mean education level of 15 years. All participants reported that they are highly motivated and eager to assist with medical research into Alzheimer's disease. Upon recruitment they attended an educational session about Alzheimer's disease in the form of a Power Point presentation, with emphasis on theories about causation of AD, including estimates of genetic susceptibility based on gender, family history, and genotype, after which they were asked to return to the research site at a later date for a blood draw. People in the intervention arm were informed a few weeks later about their APOE status. People assigned to be controls were not given this information until after the study is completed. Reactions of the subjects to APOE testing were systematically monitored by means of three follow-up structured interviews conducted by genetic counselors over the course of twelve months, and then compared with the reactions of individuals in the control group. In phase II of the project, when the four sites were involved, everyone was given their APOE status from the outset and both clinicians and counselors were involved in disclosing their APOE status to the research subjects. A subset of 65 individuals were interviewed by a small group of researchers, including myself, from Montreal.[3] These individuals volunteered to return after the completion of the basic REVEAL study to participate in hour-long open-ended interviews.

In order to carry out the "risk disclosure" portion of the study all subjects are shown a "risk curve."[4] These curves were developed by drawing on gender and age-specific incidence curves for first degree relatives of persons with AD that had already been calculated on the basis of a meta analysis of studies involving very large samples of Caucasian subjects (Green *et al.* 1997) (a modified curve is used with the Howard sample). In addition, the curves were further sub-divided by incorporating APOE genotype-specific odds ratio estimates for gender and age, reported in a second pooled analysis of 50 studies world wide (Farrer *et al.* 1997). This gives a total of 12 curves based on the six possible combinations of APOE alleles for both males and females. Risk curves for the control group were based on gender, age, and family history alone. Genetic counselors or clinicians, as the case may be, show the risk curve appropriate to each trial participant to them, and explain their estimated increased risk for AD into old age.

The graph for subjects who were assigned to the control group has two curves on it: one shows the curve for the "normal" population and the second, slightly steeper curve, represents increased risk by age for individuals who are first degree relatives of AD patients. Those people who have undergone genotyping are shown three curves on the graphs they view; the third curve represents increased risk on the basis of genotype. For individuals who are e2/3 or e3/3, their risk is increased only a small amount, on the basis of their affected relative alone. For those individuals who are ε3/4, and especially ε4/4, risk is clearly increased, but to a maximum for the 4/4s of 52 percent by age 85. Creating these risk curves entails exceedingly complex mathematical formulations (Cupples *et al.* 2004).

One justification for this research is that testing for susceptibility genes, it is argued, is likely to become increasingly common, especially in the private sector, and therefore knowledge about how people deal with risk information when it is impossible to make predictions with a high degree of confidence is urgently needed. A second justification is that to withhold information about their bodies from people is patronizing. A third justification is that in many families where someone has died of AD some members of the next generation may well believe that they have a virtually 100 percent chance of contracting the disease. If individuals can be taught that, even if they are homozygous for APOEε4, their lifetime risk for getting AD is never more than approximately 52 percent for men and 58 percent for women, then anxiety levels may well be lowered. The fourth explicit justification for the research is to create a pool of APOEε4 individuals whose blood can be used at any time to "enrich clinical trials." The majority of people who participated in the NIH study stated that they did so primarily to assist with research, rather than to learn about their own APOE status, although this information was also of considerable interest.

Interpretation of risk estimates

Results from the follow-up questionnaires indicate that people do not experience increased anxiety levels that extends much beyond the time of actually receiving their result (Larusse *et al.* 2005). By the time the open-ended interviews were carried out, more than 12 months after being told of their estimated risk, the majority of participants had transformed the estimates they had been given into accounts that "fit" with their experience of being related to someone with Alzheimer's disease, personal assessments of their own family history, and the accumulated knowledge about the disease that they had gathered from a variety of sources. In other words, risk estimates provided in the REVEAL study rarely displace "lay knowledge" that participants bring with them to the project about who in their family is particularly at risk. Rather, this "scientific" information is either nested into preexisting knowledge, simply forgotten, or even actively rejected.

Carolyn, a 52 year old psychiatric nurse from the Boston area, in contrast to most of the other subjects, clearly remembers the risk assessment she was given as part of the study. She expresses her major motivation for participating in the project as supporting her sister, who also took part in REVEAL. Carolyn is married but has no children, whereas her sister has two children, and Carolyn perceives an enormous difference in the significance of testing for the two of them:

> If Alzheimer's happens to me, it happens to me. But I would be much more concerned if I had children ... I would want to know every single thing out there. She has two kids, you know ... So when my sister learned that the testing was in Boston, I really came along for her, not so much for myself ... I mean, it's good knowledge to have for myself, but I wanted to be there for her
> ... To do it together as sisters.

Carolyn and her sister were both in the randomized group that received their APOE status. Carolyn learned she has a 3/3 genotype, whereas her sister has a 3/4 status. Carolyn's experience as a caregiver contributed to her response to her sister's results:

> In all honesty, I try not to think about it, because when I think about it I think about what I went through with my dad. I really don't want to think about going through it with her, you know.

When asked specifically about her reaction to her own results, Carolyn responded:

> I didn't think one way or the other when I found out my risk factor.

But she adds,

> Knowledge is power. I really believe that. I mean, I don't think you can necessarily change your destiny, but certainly to go through life with your eyes only half open doesn't help you at all.

However Carolyn remains unsure of what kinds of actions such power might motivate:

> I think (REVEAL) provides useful information ... Just don't ask me how I would use it.... I honestly don't know.

Perhaps this response by Caroline is a partial answer as to why, a year after testing, nearly 75 percent of the participants had forgotten, mixed up or were confused about their risk estimates. This is particularly noteworthy when 91 percent of the informants stated that "wanting to know" their genotype was a major motivation for participation in the REVEAL study. And they would recommend that their friends and relatives also go through such testing.

Although most could not recall their risk estimates accurately, nearly half had retained the gist of the information – usually they were able to recall if they have a "good" or "bad" gene. Among the four people who were given the highest risk estimates, the homozygous ε4s, three were able to recall their genotype, and the fourth remembered that she has the "bad genes." She said, when interviewed: "I'm still totally confused, although I know I have two of them, whatever those bad things are." Another individual, also a double ε4, although she remembers that her increased lifetime risk is not quite 60 percent (some of which she has lived through) nevertheless remains convinced that she will without a doubt get the disease, as she already believed before she entered the study. This individual has seven affected relatives, and no doubt this contributes to her certainty about her future, despite what she has been taught about AD risk in REVEAL.

The single African American who is homozygous for ε4 has only one affected relative, her mother. Pearl is able to recall her genotype, and has a rough idea of her increased risk over the coming years; however she says that she knew about this risk anyway because of her "blood" (meaning her family history) and adds, "really, it's all up to God, you know." She is pleased she was tested, and angry with her sisters because they simply "brushed off" her result, as she puts it. Pearl was hoping REVEAL would "prove" that she wouldn't get AD, but now she is back in God's hands. She says she was anxious while going through the study, but that this anxiety let up quite quickly once she had completed all the interviews. As a result of the project she has reduced the fats in her diet and is thinking about changing her health insurance, but cannot really afford to do this. Other than her immediate family, Pearl has not told anyone about her result, not even her family doctor. She believes that what counts more than anything else is a positive attitude coupled with faith.

Other informants very clearly express their confusion about the test results:

> I would come in – from one meeting to the next, I would come in and I couldn't remember what my risk was. And to this day, I'm not 100 percent sure. But I know that it's elevated.

Another responded:

> I don't remember much … to be truthful, not much. I'm sure I have [my risk estimate] somewhere, but I don't remember where.

A third person demanded of us:

> Is it the 3/4 that's the least likely to get it? I don't even remember. But it was good news. Whatever it was.

And another stated emphatically:

Well, I know where I am at, where I stand. I can let my kids know where we stand. You know, I mean, maybe get it, maybe not.

One woman, when asked to explain more about the "bad things" replied:

I don't know. I don't know what gene it is…It's not the BRCA [a gene associated with breast cancer].

Several people found that the information provided by REVEAL conflicted with their own understanding about the future. Rebecca, 48, who learned that she has 3/3 genotype has four affected relatives. She insists:

According to that [AD test], I don't have the risk, okay? So, technically I should feel better. But I don't believe it, given my family.

Subjective experiences about memory loss appear to raise anxiety levels more so than does genotyping:

I can say that I've always felt all my life that I've had some memory issues … so, I have that little question, whether it's something that you actually had in some way even when you were very young.

… Do people wind up getting Alzheimer's who were aware of some memory problem when they were younger, and the connection hasn't been researched yet?

The concept of "blended inheritance" put forward some years ago by Martin Richards refers to a prevalent understanding among the public involving a "mixing or blending of influences from each parent," rather than one entailing a Mendelian transmission of genes (Richards 1996: 222). Such ideas stem from a long tradition of such reasoning evident as early as classical times (Turney 1995: 12). Richards suggested, in connection with single gene disorders, that the notion of blended inheritance not only conflicts with professional explanations about genetics, but also works to reduce acceptance of those same explanations, both in the classroom and the clinic (1996).

The REVEAL qualitative findings make clear that blended inheritance is, not surprisingly, also drawn on by families when confronted with inconclusive risk estimates for a complex disease such as Alzheimer's. In other words, there is a consistent tendency to identify a family member who in some way resembles the afflicted person as the individual most likely to be at risk for developing the disorder, whether individual genotypes are known or not. Anne Kerr and colleagues commented some years ago that, in effect, individuals act as their own authority about the interpretation of genomic information and this is what we also found (1998).

For example, Jane, who was given a 3/3 typing and has one affected relative comments:

My risk before 85 was just minimally more than others. To me, that made no sense ... I really believe I don't have much chance of missing it just by my genealogy. I mean ... when I look at both sides of my family, my mother's family is all – there's nothing else, just Alzheimer's. My father's side, there's no Alzheimer's. It's heart trouble and high cholesterol and high triglycerides. Well, I take after my mother.

Similarly, Laura said:

I've shown you the picture of me and my dad. We look like clones, practically, physically. And nobody's really said – I don't know whether the information is out there because I haven't read it – whether or not that makes a difference, a person's physical appearance. But I have a suspicion that it does.

When Katherine is asked if she worries about AD, she says:

Worry is a big word; does it ever cross my mind? Yes. Do I worry about it? My brother worries, and my mother worries more about my brother than me. She thinks his personality is more likely to be similar to hers than mine.

A middle-aged man, Robert, commented:

Do I think I have a higher than normal chance? Yes. Heredity. And also I'm so much like my mother, who had Alzheimer's. There's a very high likelihood that one or more of her children will have a predisposition toward it. And I would say I'm front-runner because of so many other characteristics that are very much like my mother's.

When the REVEAL interviewees discussed theories of causation, multi-causal explanations for AD were common and, despite the emphasis given to genetics throughout the trial, this did not dominate the exchanges. When asked what caused her father's illness Carolyn responded: *"I can't pinpoint any one thing."* And a 74-year-old participant, when asked in what way she believes genetics is involved in Alzheimer disease causation replied:

I think it plays a part, but I don't think that's all. I'm sure that a lot of the diet, and the health, and the exercise that we do today will prolong life and mental acuity.

A 52-year-old woman noted:

... It's a Russian roulette kind of thing. Everything's got to be working against you, whatever those factors may be. And I don't even know what. Aluminum in your teeth? You hear some of those things. I don't know.

Every one of the REVEAL participants seemed particularly receptive to what they had been taught about the uncertainty of how exactly genetics contributes to AD. The education sessions that REVEAL participants were required to attend in all probability worked to reinforce the concept of blended inheritance already in the minds of the majority of participants prior to the study. No doubt this was because it was repeatedly emphasized that the APOEε4 allele does *not* determine disease occurrence but, rather, only puts individuals at increased risk.

In summary, genetic testing for APOE status did not apparently cause increased anxiety, or only temporarily so, in part, I believe, because genomic or "science based" explanations do not displace common sense explanations. It is also evident that many individuals who believed they are at 100 percent risk for AD because of their family history were reassured that this is not the case – this applied especially to those individuals (by far the majority of participants) who were told that they do not have an ε4 allele.[5] There is, of course, a possibility that some of these people now believe they will *not* get AD, but the education session was designed to avoid this misunderstanding.

Subjectivity and susceptibility genes

The APOE gene is an effective research tool, and continued use of it by both basic scientists and population geneticists may well unravel some of the impasses with which they are currently confronted. However, it seems unlikely that much progress will be made unless serious attention is paid to epigenetics, and the way in which APOE functions in cellular contexts, in turn influenced by larger macro-environments (Jablonka and Lamb 2005; Lock 2005; Oyama *et al.* 2001; Rose 2005; Weiss and Buchanan 2003). It is highly likely that the findings from such research will show that future risk for Alzheimer's disease can never be accurately predicted on the basis of APOE testing alone, and that other environmental and/ or developmental variables may prove to have greater predictive power. Given the state of current knowledge, APOE test results are not considered to be of any use in the clinic, except on occasion to give added weight to a diagnosis of probable AD and, unless clinical trials with genotypically specific medication prove successful, this situation is unlikely to change.

The validity of the individualized risk curves and increased risk estimates that are being handed out to the REVEAL research subjects have to be questioned, given the state of current APOE knowledge. But responses of REVEAL participants suggest in any case that little if any significant changes take place with respect to their sense of identity or subjectivity as a result of the testing. Individuals do not apparently adopt genetically informed identities, nor believe their futures to be profoundly changed from what they had already envisioned, but rather hold firm to ideas already internalized about hereditary and the power of phenotypic resemblances, AD multi-causality, and the impossibility of ever being sure about the future when a stubborn disease such as AD is at issue. By far the majority of people in the REVEAL study did not appear vulnerable to media hype, nor were they fed a false optimism by taking part in the project, quite the contrary.

However, some had come into the study seeking out definitive information, only to be thwarted and disappointed.

On the other hand, given how often articles appear in the newspaper about clinics offering genetic testing (see, for example, Abraham 2005), there may well be members of the public, believing they would be acting prudently, who want to learn about their APOE status. But few, if any, would get the counseling that the REVEAL participants were given, and for them the odds of misunderstanding the probabilistic results, if they were actually informed of life-time probabilities, are very high indeed, particularly as it is clear that even with extensive counseling, people come away confused. However, given that neither family doctors, AD societies, the media, nor even internet chat rooms (Lock *et al.* in preparation) serve to heighten fears that genes determine AD, nor actively encourage testing at the present time, it seems unlikely that many people will seek out such testing even if it becomes more widely available.

When people learn about their APOE status, there is no way of knowing who among those who test positive for ε4 are likely to become demented, even within any one family. And, equally, there is no way of knowing who among the ε3s and ε2s will become demented. An acquaintance of mine, herself a genetic researcher, decided to find out the APOE status of several of her family members because two of the older generation had Alzheimer's disease. She was stunned to learn that these two family members are homozygous for ε2, the allele that is supposedly protective. Translation from population databases to individual cases is an insurmountable problem, and, given the present state of our knowledge, family history rather than APOE status is a better predictor of the future, a situation that may not change for some time.

It makes little sense, then, to socialize on the basis of shared APOE genotyping, nor is it at present possible to do so, given that testing is so limited. If, as many researchers in the Alzheimer world believe, including many geneticists, that further research will show that combinations of genes, environment, lifestyle, and other macro-variables considered together have more explanatory power than does an individual's APOE status, then it is likely that the DNA segment known as APOEε4 will never amass sufficient power, scientific or symbolic, to be a potent signifier intimately associated with dementia (however, APOE is also implicated in heart disease, and this is a different story). Clearly this gene does not captivate people the way the BRCA genes do. People are not encouraged by the medical world to be genetically prudent with respect to the APOEε4 polymorphism *because* it is a shape-shifter and unpredictable, and activism in connection with Alzheimer's disease continues to be amply generated by well established forms of biosociality: contributing financially and as research subjects to the search for medications, lobbying for better care of diagnosed patients and for improved support for home care. Countering this, beliefs that arise spontaneously in many families about blended inheritance are often divisive and not conducive to a biosocial affiliation. But then too, genotyping also has a great potential to be divisive.

Advances in molecular genetics have certainly brought about a re-problematization of life itself. But the reign of the gene as the supreme icon of this transformation is undergoing an eclipse brought about by postgenomic insights that are neither deterministic nor stable, making predictions about future confrontations with complex disease highly problematic. Given this situation, Alzheimer biosociality is likely to continue largely unchanged. Under enormous duress as a member of an Alzheimer family, individuals have little leisure to consider what might happen to themselves in 20 years time, or to their children 40 or 50 years hence. Whatever contribution genetics may have played in the unfolding tragedy is beyond all control, and worry about questionable probabilities for the future pales beside the lived experience of confronting the disease on a daily basis. It is often remembrance of times past that gives people succor and even joy, as the disease works its alarming transformations, and not premeditations about the future.

Acknowledgments

Funding for this research was provided by the Social Science and Humanities Research Council of Canada (SSHRC), grant # 205806.

The REVEAL project was supported by National Institutes of Health grants HG/AG02213 (The REVEAL Study), AG09029 (The MIRAGE Study), AG13846 (Boston University Alzheimer's disease Center), and M01 RR00533 (Boston University General Clinical Research Center.

Notes

1 This situation applies even to the so-called Mendelian genes. See, for example, with respect to Huntington's disease: Creighton *et al.* 2003.
2 My position is that the internet, rather than increasing biosociality, effectively functions in many instances to reduce human contact, although participation in chat rooms may be an exception.
3 Janalyn Prest and Stephanie Lloyd, formerly affiliated with the anthropology department at McGill University, acted as research assistants and conducted and coded most of the qualitative interviews from Phase I of the REVEAL study. Heather Lindstrom, in the Anthropology department at Case Western Reserve also conducted some interviews. Julia Freeman and Gillian Chilibeck, anthropology department, McGill University, conducted the interviews at Howard University and transcribed and coded the data.
4 See Roberts *et al.* 2005: 253 for an illustration of these graphs.
5 Results from the REVEAL quantitative interviews show that 80 percent of a sub group of people who tested 3/3 were very positive about the study, and 67 percent had lower anxiety levels about AD than they did prior to the study (LaRusse *et al.* 2005).

References

Abraham, C. (2005) "Would You Gaze Into a Genetic Crystal Ball?" *The Globe and Mail*, Quebec edn: A 1, 9–10.
Agence Nationale d'Accrédition et d'Évaluation en Santé (ANAES) (2000) "Recommandations Pratiques Pour le Diagnostic de la Maladie d'Alzheimer. Texte Des

Recommandations." *Recommandations pour la Pratique Clinique*. ANAES. Online. Available HTTP: http://www.anaes.fr/ (accessed June 2006).

Alzheimer Society of Canada (2002) Alzheimer Disease and Heredity. Online.Toronto, Alzheimer Canada. Available HTTP: http://www.alzheimer.ca/english/disease/causes-heredity.htm (accessed June 2006).

Alzheimer's Association UK (2002) "Fact Sheet" (Pamphlet).

Alzheimer's Society (2003) *Dementia Care and Research: Policy Positions*. Online. Available HTTP: www.alzheimers.org.uk (accessed June 2006).

Alzheimer's Society (2005) *Facts about Dementia*. Online. Available HTTP: http://www. alzheimers.org.uk/Facts_about_dementia/index.htm (accessed June 2006).

American College of Medical Genetics/American Society of Human Genetics Working Group on APOE and Alzheimer Disease (1995) "Statement on Use of Apolipoprotein E Testing for Alzheimer Disease," *Jama*, 274: 1627–9.

Ballenger, J. F. (2006) *Self, Senility, and Alzheimer's Disease in Modern America: A History*, Baltimore, MD: Johns Hopkins University Press.

Beach, T. G. (1987) "The History of Alzheimer's Disease: Three Debates," *Journal of the History of Medicine and Allied Sciences*, 42: 327–49.

Bertram, L. and Tanzi, R. E. (2004) "Alzheimer's Disease: One Disorder, Too Many Genes?" *Human Molecular Genetics* 13 Spec No. 1: R135–41.

Breitner, J. C. (1999) "The End of Alzheimer's Disease?" *International Journal of Geriatric Psychiatry*, 14: 577–86.

Corbo, R.M. and Scacchi, R. (1999) "Apolipoprotein E (APOE) Allele Distribution in the World. Is APOEε4 a 'Thrifty' Allele?" *Annals of Human Genetics*, 63 (Pt 4): 301–10.

Corder, E. H., Saunders, A. M., Strittmatter, W. J., Schmechel, D. E., Gaskell, P. C., Small, G. W., Roses, A. D., Haines, J. L. and Pericak-Vance, M. A. (1993) "Gene Dose of Apolipoprotein E type 4 Allele and the Risk of Alzheimer's Disease in Late Onset Families," *Science*, 261: 921–3.

Creighton, S., Almqvist, E. W., MacGregor, D., Fernandez, B., Hogg, H., Beis, J., Welch, J. P., Riddell, C., Lokkesmoe, R., Khalifa, M., Mackenzie, J., Sajoo, A., Farrell, S., Robert, F., Shugar, A., Summers, A., Meschino, W., Allingham- Hawkins, D., Chiu, T., Hunter, A., Allanson, J., Hare, H., Schween, J., Collins, L., Sanders, S., Greenberg, C., Cardwell, S., Lemire, E., Macleod, P. and Hayden, M. R. (2003) "Predictive, Pre-natal and Diagnostic Genetic Testing for Huntington's Disease: the Experience in Canada from 1987 to 2000," *Clinical Genetics*, 63: 462–75.

Cupples, L. A., Farrer, L. A., Sadovinick, A. D., Relkin, N., Whitehouse, P. and Green, R. C. (2004) "Estimating Risk Curves for First-Degree Relatives of Patients with Alzheimer's Disease: the REVEAL Study," *Genetic Medicine*, 6: 192–6.

Duster, T. (1990) *Backdoor to Eugenics*, New York and London: Routledge.

Eaton, M. L. (1999) "Surrogate Decision Making for Genetic Testing for Alzheimer Disease," *Genetic Testing*, 3: 93–7.

Farlow, M. R., He, Y., Tekin, S., Xu, J., Lane, R., Charles H. C., (2004) "Impact of APOE in Mild Cognitive Impairment," *Neurology*, 63: 1898–901.

Farrer, L. A. (2000) "Familial Risk for Alzheimer Disease in Ethnic Minorities: Non-discriminating Genes," *Archives of Neurology*, 57: 28–9.

Farrer, L. A., Cupples, L. A., Haines, J. L., Hyman, B., Kukull, W. A., Mayeux, R., Myers, R. H., Pericak-Vance, M. A., Risch, N. and Van Duijn, C. M. (1997) "Effects of Age, Sex, and Ethnicity on the Association between Apolipoprotein E Genotype and Alzheimer Disease. A Meta-Analysis." APOE and Alzheimer Disease Meta Analysis Consortium. *Jama*, 278: 1349–56.

Fox, P. (1989) "From Senility to Alzheimer's Disease: the Rise of the Alzheimer's Disease Movement," *Milbank Q*, 67: 58–102.

Franzen, J. (2001) "My Father's Brain: What Alzheimer's takes away," *The New Yorker*, 10 September: 85.

Green, R. C., Clarke, V. C., Thompson, N. J., Woodard, J. L. and Letz, R. (1997) "Early Detection of Alzheimer Disease: Methods, Markers, and Misgivings." *Alzheimer's Disease and Associated Disorders*, 11, Suppl. 5: S1–5; discussion S37–9.

Growdon, J. H. (1998) "Apolipoprotein E and Alzheimer's Disease," *Archives of Neurology*, 55: 1053–4.

Gubrium, J. F. (2000) "Narrative Practice and the Inner Worlds of the Alzheimer Disease Experience," In Whitehouse, P. J., Maurer, K. and Ballenger, J. F. (eds) *Concepts of Alzheimer Disease: Biological, Clinical, and Cultural Perspectives*, Baltimore, MD: Johns Hopkins University Press.

Hacking, I. (1986) "Making up People," In Heller, T. C., Sosna, M. and Wellerby, D. E. (eds) *Reconstructing Individualism: Autonomy, Individuality, and Self in Western Thought*, Stanford, CA: Stanford University Press.

Halpern, S. (2005) "The Gene Hunters: Closing in on the Origins of Alzheimer's Disease," *The New Yorker*: 84–93.

Hardy, J. (1997) "The Alzheimer Family of Diseases: Many Etiologies, One Pathogenesis?" *Proc Natl Acad Sci USA*, 94: 2095–7.

Health Canada (2001) "Genetic Testing for Late Onset Diseases: In-Depth Thematic Analysis of Policy and Jurisdictional Issues." Ministry of Supply and Services.

Holstein, M. (1997) "Alzheimer's Disease and Senile Dementia, 1885–1920: An Interpretive History of Disease Negotiation," *Journal of Aging Studies*, 11: 1–13.

Hyman, B. T., Gomez-Isla, T., Briggs, M., Chung, H., Nichols, S., Kohout, F. and Wallace, R. (1996) "Apolipoprotein E and Cognitive Change in an Elderly Population," *Annals of Neurology*, 40: 55–66.

Ince, P. G. (2001) "Random, Chance, or Hazard?" *J Clin Pathol*, 54: 254.

Jablonka, E. and Lamb, M. J. (2005) *Evolution in Four Dimensions: Genetic, Epigenetic, Behavioral, and Symbolic Variation in the History of Life*, Cambridge, MA: MIT Press.

Journal of the American Medical Association (2001) American College of Medical Genetics Position Statement: Genetic Testing for Late-Onset Alzheimer's Disease. Online. AGS Ethics Committee. Available from: http://www.americangeriatrics.org/products/positionpapers/gen_test.shtml (accessed May 2004).

Katzman, R. (1976) "Editorial: The Prevalence and Malignancy of Alzheimer Disease. A Major Killer," *Archives of Neurology*, 33: 217–8.

Kerr, A., Cunningham-Burley, S. and Amos, A. (1998) "The New Genetics and Health: Mobilizing Lay Expertise," *Public Understanding of Science*, 7: 41–60.

Khachaturian, Z. S. (1997) "Plundered Memories," *The Sciences*, 37: 21–5.

Kier, F. J. and Molinari, V. (2003) "'Do-it-yourself' Dementia Testing: Issues Regarding an Alzheimer's Home Screening Test," *Gerontologist*, 43: 295–301.

Korovaitseva, G. I., Shcherbatykh, T. V., Selezneva, N. V., Gavrilova, S. I., Golimbet, V. E., Voskresenskaia, N. I. and Rogachev, E. I. (2001) "Genetic Association Between the Apolipoprotein E [ApoE] Gene Alleles and Various Forms of Alzheimer's Disease," *Human Genetics*, 37: 422–2.

LaRusse, S., Roberts, J. S., Marteau, T. M., Katzen, H., Linnenbringer, E. L., Barber, M., Whitehouse, P., Quaid, K., Brown, T., Green, R. C. and Relkin, N. R. (2005) "Genetic

Susceptibility Testing Versus Family History-Based Risk Assessment: Impact on Perceived Risk of Alzheimer Disease," *Genetic Medicine*, 7: 48–53.

Latour, B. (1993) *We Have Never Been Modern*, Cambridge, MA: Harvard University Press.

Lock, M. (2005) "Eclipse of the Gene and the Return of Divination," *Current Anthroplogy*, 46: S47–S70.

Lock M., Lloyd S. and Prest J., (2006) "Genetic Susceptibility and Alzheimer's Disease: The Penetrance and Uptake of Genetic Knowledge," in Leibing, A. and Cohen, L. (eds) *Thinking about Dementia: Culture, Loss and the Anthropology of Senility*, Piscataway, NJ: Rutgers University Press.

Lock, M., Freeman, J., Sharples, R. and Lloyd, S. (2006) "When it Runs in the Family: Putting Susceptibility Genes in Perspective," *Public Understanding of Science*, 15: 277–300.

Lock, M., Freeman, J., Padowsky, M. Chilibeck, G. and Beveridge, B. (in press) "Susceptibility Genes and the Question of Embodied Identity."

McConnell, L. M., Koenig, B. A., Greely, H. T. and Raffint, A. (1998) "Genetic Testing and Alzheimer Disease: Has the Time Come?" *Nature Medicine*, 4: 757–9.

Moss, L. (2003) *What Genes Can't Do*, Cambridge, MA: MIT Press.

Myers, R. H., Schaeffer, E. J., Wilson, P. W., D'Agostino, R., Ordovas, J. M., Espino, A., Au, R., White, R. F., Knoefel, J. E., Cobb, J. L., McNulty, K. A., Beiser, A. and Wolf, P. A. (1996) "Apolipoprotein E Epsilon4 Association with Dementia in a Population-based Study: The Framingham Study," *Neurology*, 46: 673–7.

Nelkin, D. and Tancredi, L. R. (1989) *Dangerous Diagnostics: the Social Power of Biological Information*, New York: Basic Books.

Novas, C. and Rose, N. (2000) "Genetic Risk and the Birth of the Somatic Individual," *Economy and Society*, 29: 485–513.

Novek S. (2006) "The Struggle for Symbolic Understanding: A Qualitative Analysis of Caregivers' Experiences with Dementia," unpublished thesis, McGill University.

Offit, K., Groeger, E., Turner, S., Wadsworth, E. A. and Weiser, M. A. (2004) "The 'Duty to Warn' A Patient's Family Members about Hereditary Disease Risks," *Jama*, 292: 1469–73.

Oyama, S., Griffiths, P. E. and Gray, R. D. (2001) *Cycles of Contingency: Developmental Systems and Evolution*, Cambridge, MA: MIT Press.

Rabinow, P. (1994) "The Third Culture," *History of the Human Sciences*, 7: 53–64.

Relkin, N. R., Kwon, Y. J., TSAI, J. and Gandy's, S. (1996) "The National Institute on Aging/Alzheimer's Association Recommendations on the Application of Apolipoprotein E genotyping to Alzheimer's Disease," *Ann N Y Acad Sci*, 802: 149–76.

Richards, M. (1996) "Lay and Professional Knowledge of Genetics and Inheritance," *Public Understanding of Science*, 5: 217–30.

Risner, M. E., Saunders, A. M., Altman, J. F., Ormandy, G. C., Craft, S., Foley, I. M., Zwartau-Hind, M. E., Hosford, D. A. and Roses, A. D. (2006) "Efficacy of Rosiglitazone in a Genetically Defined Population with Mild-to-Moderate Alzheimer's Disease," *Pharmacogenomics Journal*, 6(2): 246–54.

Roberts, J. S., Cupples, A., Relkin, N. R., Whitehouse, P. and Green, R. (2005) "Genetic Risk Assessment for Adult Children of People with Alzheimer's Disease: the Risk Evaluation and Education for Alzheimer Disease (REVEAL) Study," *Journal of Geriatric Psychiatry and Neurology*, 18: 250–5.

Rose, S. P. R. (2005) *The Future of the Brain: the Promise and Perils of Tomorrow's Neuroscience*, Oxford and New York: Oxford University Press.

Roses, A. D. (1998) "Apolipoprotein E and Alzheimer's Disease: The Tip of the Susceptibility Iceberg." *Annals of the New York Academy of Sciences*, 855: 738–43.

Saunders, A. M. (2000) "Apolipoprotein E and Alzheimer Disease: an Update on Genetic and Functional Analyses." *Journal Neuropathology and Experimental Neurology*, 59: 751–8.

Selkoe, D. J. (2002) "The Pathophysiology of Alzheimer's Disease," in Scinto, L.F.M. and Daffner, K.R. (eds) *Early Diagnosis of Alzheimer's Disease*, Totowa, NJ: Humana Press.

Silverman, J. M., Smith, C. J., Marin, D. B., Mohs, R. C. and Propper, C. B. (2003) "Familial Patterns of Risk in Very Late-Onset Alzheimer Disease," *Archives of General Psychiatry*, 60: 190–7.

Sleegers, K., Roks, G., Theuns, J., Aulchenko, Y. S., Rademakers, R., Cruts, M., van Gool, W. A., van Broeckhoven, C., Heutink, P., Oostra, B. A., van Swieten, J. C. and van Duijn, C.M. (2004) "Familial Clustering and Genetic Risk for Dementia in a Genetically Isolated Dutch Population," *Brain*, 127: 1641–9.

St George-Hyslop, P. H. (2000) "Molecular Genetics of Alzheimer's Disease," *Biological Psychiatry*, 47: 183–99.

Templeton, A. R. (1998) "The Complexity of the Genotype-Phenotype Relationship and the Limitations of Using Genetic 'Markers' at the Individual Level," *Science in Context*, 11: 373–89.

Tilley, L., Morgan, K. and Kalsheker, N. (1998) "Genetic Risk Factors in Alzheimer's Disease," *Molecular Pathology*, 51: 293–304.

Turney, J. (1995) "The Public Understanding of Genetics – Where next?" *European Journal of Genetics and Society*, 1: 5–22.

Weiss, K. and Buchanan, A. V. (2003) "Evolution by Phenotype: a Biomedical Perspective," *Perspectives in Biology and Medicine*, 46: 159–82.

Whitehouse, P. J. (2001) "The End of Alzheimer Disease," *Alzheimer's Disease and Associated Disorders*, 15: 59–62.

Zick, C. D., Mathews, C. J., Roberts, J. S., Cook-Deegan, R., Pokorski, R. J. and Green, R. C. (2005) "Genetic Testing for Alzheimer's Disease and its Impact on Insurance Purchasing Behavior," *Health Affairs (Millwood)*, 24: 483–90.

4 Biology, sociality and reproductive modernity in Ecuadorian *in-vitro* fertilization

The particulars of place

Elizabeth F. S. Roberts

Introduction

Late nineteenth- and early twentieth-century Europe and North America have been characterized as the "age of the womb" because of the "epidemic" of modern upper class female nervous disorders during this period (Davis and Low 1989: 2). Whenever in Ecuador I feel like I am living amidst an ongoing "age of the womb," but one with a dizzying array of new technical and surgical options to cure the feminine afflictions of modernity. Young, childless, middle-class Ecuadorian women seem to have all undergone some sort of reproductive surgery or treatment (laparoscopy, fibroid removal, or had intensive hormonal therapy), usually for physical problems that remained somewhat undefined. Later on, pregnancy intensifies their commitment to bodily invasion as they prepared for their inevitable cesarean section. The young women undergoing these surgeries and treatments are often *sure* that they cannot have children because of their reproductive troubles. In the context of these failed bodies, the arrival of assisted reproductive technologies in Ecuador, such as *in-vitro* fertilization (IVF), did not produce the expectation that their bodies would fail (although they have surely exacerbated it). Anticipatory infertility was already well in place among many Ecuadorian women since it is assumed that a modern woman's body is likely to experience some sort of reproductive malfunction throughout her lifetime. For *in-vitro* fertilization (IVF) patients in Ecuador, with whom I have conducted research since 2000, IVF is an achievement of sorts, a sign of what I call *reproductive modernity* – a class based norm that entails financial sacrifice and the bodily markers of modern biological dysfunction.[1]

IVF is one of many bio-medical operations and interventions that produce social status through biological identity in Ecuador, however we should not necessarily take the participation of Ecuadorian women in reproductive modernity as examples of biosociality as described by Paul Rabinow (Rabinow 1996). The task of this volume is to empirically examine the concept of biosociality. To that end, my research on IVF in Ecuador places a limit on the concept. This does not mean I am arguing with the validity of biosociality as a concept applied to contemporary identity-making practices shaped by novel biological knowledge in Europe and North America. Instead, by describing a site where biotechnologies have not, at least yet, reshaped the biological or the social, in the same way as in Europe and North America, we have an opportunity to establish the relevance of the analytic concept to a particular time and place. We can ask, what assemblages of concepts and normed bodies produce a configuration that social scientists can categorize as biosociality, and what might not? Limiting the concept of biosociality, situates it, makes it of a place and set of conditions, preventing the tendency to universalize concepts and thus ignore the specific circumstances that shape how norms are produced in the world.

IVF in Ecuador

In 1992 the Ecuadorian news media proudly heralded the birth of Ecuador's first IVF baby, and since then local media coverage of assisted reproduction has continued unabated, touting Ecuador's ability to keep pace with other modern countries through the techno-scientific production of children. As of 2004 there were nine active IVF clinics in Ecuador with more in the planning stages, this number in an impoverished nation of less than 12 million inhabitants. By my estimate these nine clinics conduct a total of 350 to 400 IVF cycles a year. This constitutes a very small percentage of the total population, but the ubiquity of popular media coverage about these clinics indicates that there is a general knowledge about the availability of IVF. Indeed, whenever I told middle class Ecuadorians about my work most had heard of the process and even knew someone who had undergone the treatment.[2]

Ecuador has some of the leading indicators of poor health in Latin America, as well as a much-noted shortage of doctors in the public sector (CEPAR 2000). The total number of doctors per inhabitants in Ecuador has almost quadrupled in the last twenty years and continues to rise as doctors are increasingly drawn to the private sector. Officially, most Ecuadorians have access to free or low cost health services, through either the Ministry of Public Health through service in the armed forces, or through formal sector employment. However the public health system, especially the services provided by the Ministry of Public Health, is underfunded, terribly managed, and corrupt. As a result patients are treated abysmally: there are few supplies, buildings are crumbling, and iatrogenic infection is common. The Ecuadorian state spends only 2 percent of its annual budget on public health. In Latin America only Haiti spends less (Vos *et al.*).

Due to the retraction of social welfare spending by the state and the related expansion of the for-profit health sector, patients of all economic levels are quite accustomed to paying out of pocket in order to avoid publicly funded medical care (Vos *et al.* 2004). Private sector medicine in Ecuador is flourishing, a free-marketer's dream, with ubiquitous advertisements for every sort of medical specialist at all price ranges blanketing the cityscapes. The World Health Organization estimates that in 2002 64 percent of all health spending in Ecuador came from private sources. Of those expenditures 88.4 percent were directly out of pocket from individual and family household incomes (WHO 2005). Almost all private sector medicine offers something beyond what Ecuadorians can expect in the public sector. The most expensive private clinics have the latest technologies and services, but even the more moderately priced and cheapest private clinics provide a level of personalized patient care that is impossible to find in public sector healthcare.

In their global distribution, assisted reproductive biotechnologies are often understood in relation to discourses of "modernity," "progress," "development," and "catching up." In Ecuador, science and technologies, such as assisted reproductive technologies, are seen as quintessential building blocks of modernity. Local news reports on Ecuadorian IVF clinics and its practitioners are mobilized as a symbol of pride in the progress of private sector medicine (Bustamante 1989; Gomez 1991). However the pride surrounding IVF had little to do with pride in the nation state, which is commonly seen as ongoing failure, but instead pride at the fact that there are individual, modern, Ecuadorian, doctor entrepreneurs offering these technical innovations.

Biosociality

In Paul Rabinow's essay "Artificiality and Enlightenment: From Sociobiology to Biosociality," he described how bio-technological advances including genomics had generated new understandings of the biological as shaped by the social. Rabinow argued that the *biological* had recently changed from fixed to malleable through cultural practices.

> If sociobiology is culture constructed on the basis of a metaphor of nature, then in biosociality nature will be modeled on culture understood as practice. Nature will be known and remade throughout technique and will finally become artificial, just as culture becomes natural.
>
> (Rabinow 1996: 99)

The *social*, in biosociality involved the creation of new identities and groupings around this *newly* malleable biology. Thus he predicted:

> It is not hard to imagine groups formed around the chromosome 17, locus 16,256, site 654,376 allele variant with a guanine substitution … These are new biological groupings that will crosscut, partially supersede, and eventually redefine the older categories [of race and sex] in ways that are well worth monitoring.
>
> (Rabinow 1996: 102)

Rabinow's emphasis on the novelty of these groupings refers back to his discussion of the novelty of biological malleability. As he is careful to point out, these groupings do not so much replace older biological groupings like race and sex, as they redefine them. This point is crucial to my argument about the limits of biosociality. I contend that the concept should not be applied to every social grouping formed around biological identity, or disease status, if these groupings do not involve an emergent shift in biological thinking towards the malleable. However, my focus on the biological side of biosociality is not how the term is most commonly deployed.

For the most part, scholars who have harnessed biosociality to their own projects have focused more on the social half of biosociality. They describe activist patient groups cohered around a problematic biological status, as they interact with formal institutions such as state ministries, or pharmaceutical firms. Nikolas Rose and Carlos Novas emphasized the sociality of biosociality (and less the new malleability of biology), when they noted that biosociality is not necessarily "new," as "collectivities formed around a biological conception of a shared identity – have a long history that predate recent developments in bio-medicine and genomics" (Rose and Novas 2005: 442). For Rose and Novas the novelty of biosociality does not come from these groupings nor new biologically plastic epistemologies, but from the newly intensified "scientific and medical knowledge" of their bodies that these activist groups possess. Likewise, Rayna Rapp described biosociality as the "forging of collective identity under the emergent categories of biomedicine and allied sciences" (Rapp 1999: 302).[3]

Veena Das also focused on the social side of biosociality, by defining biosociality as "the forming of associational communities to influence state policy and science" (Das 2001). However, Das argues that the concept does not work particularly well in locations like India where most groups lack bio-capital, "the capacity of a group to use social capital for dealing with biological conditions" (Das 2001: 2). In Das's research in poor Delhi neighborhoods, she found that, in managing stigmatizing conditions like facial disfigurements, families do interact with the state. According to Das, these family groupings indicate new patterns of sociality around biological conditions in India through "new alignments of the domestic sphere with the state, against social pressures generated by local communities" (Das 2001: 3). These groupings are not biosocial though, because biosociality presumes "the individual as the subject of a liberal political regime, which Das finds foreign to the types of socialities at work for the urban poor in India" (Das 2001: 3). These new "alignments between family and state" embody a "politics of domesticity, which involve connected body selves" not liberal individuals (Das 2001: 3).

Like Das, my research demonstrates that we should question the relevance of applying the concept of biosociality to every contemporary practice that involves emergent biological status. Similar to Das's description of poor neighborhoods in Delhi, *the social* in Ecuador is not the same as it is in Europe and North America. Ecuador's colonial history and current international status as a chronically unstable democracy, with little civil society, has produced a very different concept of the social (Gerlach 2003; Whitten 2003). Thus in Ecuador there are no activist patient groups that advocate for themselves as liberal subjects in relation to a state. My larger point however, is that biosociality is also less applicable to Ecuador, in regards to *the biological*, itself. In Ecuador the biological has not historically signified the universal fixity that has been common to North America and Europe. Biology in Ecuador and throughout much of the Andes and Latin America has tended to be less essential than malleable. Thus one of biosociality's two most salient characteristics, the emergence of nature as "artificial" able to be "remade throughout technique" is not necessarily new to the Andes.

Sociality and citizenship

In Ecuador, associational groups do not coalesce around new biological identities, although as I argue below class membership is intimately tied to biological status. The absence of biosocial collectivities has to do with the devalued nature of citizenship in Ecuador, and the retraction of the social welfare sector of the state. In parsing biosociality, a few scholars of Europe have tied the concept to citizenship, which exemplifies why the concept has little analytical relevance to Ecuador. For Rose and Novas becoming worthy of "biological citizenship" entails the biosociality of self-prudent yet enterprising individuals actively optimizing their lives (Rose and Novas 2005). Adriana Petryana's work on the Ukraine also connects biosociality to citizenship in describing how ex-Chernobyl workers are able to make demands upon a new state through their biological status as sufferers of radiation sickness (Petryna 2002). These formulations of biosociality and citizenship entail a state (no matter how privatized) that is assumed to be a stable entity that can distribute desirable social welfare benefits. This is not the case in Ecuador.

The leftist, populist military junta of the 1970s decentered elites from the Ecuadorian state (Gerlach 2003). The junta ended in 1984, but the subsequent discovery of oil in the Amazon, leading to short lived economic boom then subsequent economic bust, has marked "less the return of the economic elites to controlling the state and more their success in assuring that the state would no longer control them" (Krupa 2004: 14). Confidence in government in Ecuador, among all classes, is extremely low especially after the recent toppling of the eighth president in less than eight years. Currently status has everything to do with one's ability to maneuver around the state and the law, or as one IVF practitioners, told me, "pass above it." Status is not derived from one's ability to make public demands upon government offices. Social welfare programs are all seen as inferior to private health care, education, and security. It is the poor who use public services and indigenous groups who form social movements to make political demands on the state, not the middle classes or elites. Of course from the point of view of state actors there might be benefits to being considered an inferior provider in this time of IMF mandated austerity measures and decreased social spending.

The state remains a potent bureaucratic force in the everyday lives of those who need public services. In Ecuador, prosaic tasks which I never gave much thought to in the United States, such as paying bills, replacing a lost driver's license, entering a public swimming pool, registering for public education, and using public medical care represent an absurdly large drain on the temporal and emotional resources of the poorer economic sector. These people cannot "pass above" these requirements, as they do not have employees to stand in line for them, cannot afford *tramitadores* to deal with the required paperwork, and do not have the resources to avoid them all together. Deborah Poole argues that, in the Andes, these sites of interface, where the state demands payment or distributes services are where poor and indigenous citizen subjects are made to learn the "gap between membership and belonging" (Poole 2004: 17). The multitudes are disciplined to the inequities of standing in line for unequal resources while the connected jump ahead or are ushered in to back rooms, or don't require these services at all. To stand in line is to assume the position of the masses, whose only recourse is the law. Those who do not have to interact with the state in Ecuador are elite by definition, and can make their own forms of freedoms outside the law. Forming a collectivity to make demands around one's biological status would make little sense in this context.

IVF patients in Ecuador do not desire recognition from the state. They have not banded together around their status as infertile, as they have in the United States through organizations like RESOLVE, a self-help support group and consumer rights organization that advocates for the infertile (a newly medicalized category) in order to influence public policy and the insurance industry (Becker 2000). Infertility patients have no reason to cohere as a group to advocate for themselves in terms of treatment or service given that state recognition would get them nothing. What's more, socializing in this way would confer inferior class status through the act of asking for inferior services. A very few Ecuadorian IVF patients expressed a desire to talk to others undergoing similar experiences with childlessness, while most told me that they would not be interested in this type of socializing. I must emphasize that reluctance to socialize around childlessness did not only come from the stigma associated with infertility. While infertility was a painful subject for many of those involved in IVF, I found that the use of IVF to fix infertility was often a source of pride, not something that was kept a secret from family, friends or children produced through the procedure. No one imagined however, that it would be useful to have a larger collective identity to advocate for resources for their infertility.

In addition, only a very few of the patients I encountered engaged in the sort of educated consumerist behavior I was so accustomed to in the United States. One women, Tatiana, an accountant and department supervisor at a bank did actively consume information about IVF. She was the most "informed" IVF patient I met in Ecuador. Tatiana avidly read Spanish language internet accounts of other women's experiences of IVF from Buenos Aires, Miami, and Mexico City. She would bring these accounts to her appointments so she could refer to them while she waited. No other IVF patient, except one, ever mentioned learning about the experience of IVF through web sites or magazines. This other patient, Lourdes, undergoing IVF for the third time, explained to me that she read internet accounts of IVF during her first cycle. But they made her more "anxious" to know about other people's experiences and opinions so she stopped.

Like Lourdes, the majority of patients in Ecuadorian IVF clinics did not fashion themselves as educated consumers of IVF, and they did not feel the need to be in charge of their own care. They left that to the experts – the doctors who they trusted. Repeatedly, patients told me that what they looked for in a doctor was professionalism, which for them meant "charisma" and "humanity," not higher success rates, or the latest procedures. Patients expected to be able to call doctors and other staff at all times of the day or night on their cell phone or at home and receive in-depth attention. Patients expected their doctors to treat them like daughters, which doctors did, usually greeting them with kisses and endearments, patting them before and after procedures. In this realm doctors and God were not all that differentiated. The halls of the clinics were lined with photos of babies, and also commemorative engraved plaques of thanks to the clinic director, sometimes calling him "our scientific papa." These plaques were the same as the ones found at religious shrines throughout Ecuador left in gratitude to God for miraculous healing. Patients enjoyed the benefits of patienthood under the care of physicians who took a keen personalized interest in their care, a form of patienthood impossible to find in public sector medicine. Thus patienthood in Ecuador did not involve the social – group cohesion or antagonistic activism towards the medical establishment in relation to larger administering institutions like the state. It did not involve a new understanding of the biological either.

Biological malleability

From the late nineteenth century *the biological* in Western Europe and North America came to be scientifically and popularly viewed as determinate of characteristics that could not be changed by human effort or the environment (Leyes Stepan 1982; Strathern 1992). Biology also came to be understood as universal, in the sense that biological systems function the same everywhere (Gordon 1988; Lock and Gordon 1988). In the last two decades many biologists have become increasingly fascinated with the malleability of biology through genomics (Keller 2000), and as Rabinow described, popular understandings of the biological in North America and Europe are now changing in tandem with these new biological modes of thought. These recent shifts towards a more plastic biology might not have the same sort of popular impact in Ecuador however, where, as in much of Latin America, biology has historically been understood as malleable. One of the main reasons for this biological malleability in Latin America had to do with the history of state formation and race politics, a history made visible in IVF clinics.

In Latin America the question of race is played out very differently from in Europe. European nations were built through ideologies of exclusion, fears of degeneracy, and purification, in the name of those "native to the soil." But for Latin American, nation-building elites, race could not serve the same purificatory function as it did in Europe or else it would have excluded the majority of the populace, who had little claim to purity of white blood or alternatively to the soil (Foucault 1990; Stoler 1995). Thus, in Latin America racial policies emphasized miscegenation towards the goal of whitening, through national myths of *mestizaje* – the mixture of Indian and Spanish races. Unlike European states who supervised sexuality to prevent degeneracy through racial mixing, the sexual supervisions of liberal reformers in Latin America often involved assimilating/exterminating Indians through sexual congress (Cadena 2000; Sommers 2002; Wade 1993).

Mestizaje involved (and still involves) a different epistemological stance towards biology than popular forms of biological determinism in Europe. Historians of nineteenth- and twentieth-century Latin America have noted that biological and racial thinking was less about singular determinism than malleability, where the "environment," took on a large role in shaping people bodies and behaviors. Nancy Leyes Stepan's work on the early twentieth-century eugenic movements in Latin America demonstrates how French imported, neo-Lamarckian thought, which emphasized "slow purposeful adaptation to changes in the environment," prevailed over "harder" Darwinian and Mendelian ideas about inheritance (Leyes Stepan 1991: 68). Darwinian thought was less appealing in Latin America with its focus on random variation, and the brute struggle for survival, models of "change that seemed to take all design out of the universe" in theories of racial betterment (Leyes Stepan 1991: 68). At several points, eugenic congresses in Latin America voted to ignore North American and European eugenic mandates, because of the immutability and determinism of their racial thinking (Leyes Stepan 1991).

Today in Latin America the concept of race is often tied to ideas about custom, tradition, environment, all more pliant modes of racial thinking than in North America and Europe. The large scholarship on racial and ethnic categories in the Andes has demonstrated that the racial category of *mestizo* is a particularly shifting identity (Colloredo-Mansfeld 1998; Mallon 1996; Orlove 1998; Poole 1997; Stutzman 1981). Mary Weistmantel writing about race in the Andes describes one version of this biological malleability among highland indigenous people in the central Andes, who "insisted that race was a physical reality, irreducible to ethnicity or social class – and yet spoke matter-of-factly about neighbors who changed their race during their lifetime" (Weismantel 2001: 191). Weismantel contrasts this way of thinking about biology and race to Andean urbanites who insisted on the importance of fixed biological connection. I found, however, that many urban mestizos involved with IVF shared in the view that race and biology were not fixed, but rather pliable and local classifications.

Egg donation

Ecuador's history of nation building in a land of "racial impurity" is deeply inscribed in contemporary practices of anonymous egg donation in Ecuadorian IVF clinics. IVF practitioners, and the vast majority of patients, thought of themselves as *mestizos* and their approach to classifying anonymous donors used racial idioms of *mestizaje*, in which mixture whitens offspring. The stated goal of these practitioners was to match patients with gamete donors as much "like them" as possible, but when an exact match was not possible, lighter was assumed to be better. However, determining which donor was the best match for a patient, often involved characteristics like class and social type, which were both seen as intrinsic in the *race* of donors.

During my observations at one clinic, Dr. Molina, an IVF clinic director, instituted a more "systematic" way of matching egg donors to recipients. He showed me his Excel spreadsheet on the computer that had columns for race and skin color. When I asked him about the difference between *mestiza clara* and *mestizo oscuro*, two categories in the race column, he explained that it "is difficult to determine, there are so many types of races here." He pointed to me and declared that I was *blanco*/white. Continuing, he described how people like him are *mestiza clara* (light mixed), then there are people who are *mestiza oscura* (dark mixed) – a classically evolutionary racial order, from lighter to darker. We moved to the next column – skin color. *Clara* signified clear/light or white, followed by *triguena clara* (light brown, olive complected), *triguena oscura* (medium brown), then *negro* and *oriental*, both which seemed to have little to do with skin color. We had come back to race again.

Dr. Molina identified himself, as *trigueno claro*, but added it "is very difficult to pick a donor by skin color and race." Then Dr. Molina lowered his voice and told me that *trigueno* was actually his secret key. People who are *trigueno oscuro* are more Indian in dress and behavior. His voice got lower still and then he switched to English. He told me he observed people carefully and people who look more Indian or more mixed are *trigueno oscuro*. *Trigueno claro* was really "people like us," "our social class." Dr. Molina's typology used the language of race to determine appropriate egg donors. But "in secret" he used markers of class to make the different determination of race. Dr. Molina's key provided him with a means to differentiate people with the same skin color but whose social class makes them a different race, which then serves to distinguish skin color.

In addition to the fact that race was determined in egg donation by taking into account factors that for North Americans and Europeans are not biological, in Ecuadorian egg donation genetic identity was not seen determining the whole truth of biological relatedness either. For many IVF patients, eggs were like a small organ or physical substance that women needed to conceive. In determining motherhood in egg donor situations the gestating mother's blood was usually of greater importance. The question was whose blood feeds the child *in utero*? I was with Linda, a laboratory biologist at another clinic one morning as she talked with Martiza and her husband Franklin. Obviously Franklin had something on his mind because he lingered after Martiza's daily hormone shots were administered. He finally blurted out a question to Linda, asking her if they used donor eggs would any of his wife "be in the child." Linda began her answer by explaining that genetically a child would be the egg donor's and his own. The donor would give the genetic information, "the [intended] mother transmits nothing." But, she added,

> The mother would exchange blood with the baby. If the woman gets pregnant there is an interchange of blood, and the child already looks like the father because it's his sperm. In fact children always look like the family that raises them. It's like adoption. It's incredible. Every one thinks they look the same. They have similar characteristics over time.

Franklin seemed satisfied with this answer and left. For Franklin, Linda had made blood and genes into countervailing forces of inheritance, where the exchange of characteristics through blood was preeminent over the transmission of information through genes. Linda's kinship reckoning deployed a mode of relatedness that recognizes exchanges of care and cultivation *in utero* as robust markers of biological connection, and her remarks about adoption evoked contemporary Andean understandings of relatedness as actualized through care, level of education and custom. In the case of egg donation the blood of a woman's uterus provides an environment of care and feeding through blood that easily overrode genes as the sole arbiter of relatedness.

Emotions, IVF and local biology

Women's experiences of their bodies as they underwent IVF did not always correspond to common North American universalist versions of biology either. In the early 1990s I conducted research with IVF patients, surrogate mothers, and egg and sperm donors in the United States (Roberts 1998a, 1998b). The hormones used throughout IVF cycles and the emotional states they caused were a common topic of conversation among all of these participants in assisted conception. Throughout this investigation, however, I never specifically analyzed the role of hormones; perhaps because "hormone talk" was so ubiquitous it was unnoticeable. This fact only became noteworthy to me after spending time with Ecuadorian women who did not put hormones to this rhetorical or experiential use.

Similar to the United States most women undergoing IVF in Ecuador narratized IVF as emotionally tumultuous, but in Ecuador this tumult usually arose from a complex set of factors involving the disruption of ordinary life by infertility and its treatments, and the struggle to maintain familial obligations. Hormones were on occasion used to explain depressive states but for the most part they were only invoked in conjunction with the social environment of the woman using them. Although irritability, nerves, and stress were commonly described by women in their IVF accounts, when I asked these women about hormones directly, the most standard response was a blank look, or something like Roxana's reply as she was undergoing IVF for a second time:

> No, in me, no. Nothing affected me. Because the doctor told me that it might put me in a bad mood. But to me it wasn't that. I had this feeling that if I was going to get pregnant that nothing was important. I suffered a little from the injections, when they put them in the *pompies* [slang for buttocks]. How strange it was. That hurt yes, but moods, no. What did give me pain was a headache, but what they said would affect me did not affect me. Everything hurt and the blood tests are constant. And sometimes I think that because so many things have come to me at once. It was a mood I had already. I don't know if the hormones did anything. There were many things … What's more I am also studying. With all the things together – the house – the husband, there are always problems.

Roxana viewed her moods around IVF as indicative of a larger set of problems even though her particular doctor prepared her to view them as solely biological in origin. IVF meant being subjected to a somewhat arduous bodily process. For Roxana, undergoing IVF entailed time away from other obligations, revolving around school, work, and her husband. Like Roxana, the vast majority of Ecuadorian IVF patients rarely relied on deterministic biological agents like hormones to explain their moods, but instead used a sort of emotional physiology for understanding their experience and the results of IVF.

In the United States emotional states are much more likely to be attributed to hormones as biological agents with unvarying universal effects (Oudshoorn 1994). Women in North America often characterize their use of infertility hormones as the primary biological cause for the intense emotional states they experience during their cycles. One woman undergoing IVF in the United States explained:

> Lupron is like going into madness. I get on Lupron and I get this agitated depression, really severe. I have never felt so suicidal in my life … You kind of know on some level it's just the chemicals. I'm not looking forward to it, especially with the agitation on top of it … . So in some ways, the Lupron is just this little shot in your thigh, it seems so benign. But it's not. The depression seems like such a common response to Lupron.
>
> (Becker 2000: 88)

For this woman biological hormones produce fixed emotional effects. She must grapple with the fact that Lupron is "just" a chemical, but a chemical that unambiguously generates something akin to madness. Nevertheless she can take comfort in the fact that in the United States this response is common ground for women undergoing IVF. In North America hormones are biological agents that have predictable responses in most women. Certainly in longer conversations with North American women about their experience of IVF, women add other explanatory layers to account for their emotional/physiological states beyond hormones (Becker 2000). But it is incontrovertible that in the United States hormones are often put to work as singular agents of emotional instability in IVF. In the United States hormones act as cultural shorthand for expressing emotional disturbance, a shorthand that allows for certain interpretations of experience to be emphasized over others. The biological becomes inescapable. The prevalence of hormonal thinking is indicative of a particular biological epistemology very different from that found in Ecuador where interpretations of emotional upheaval are immediately connected to more than one agent, and are usually thought to be environmentally induced.

Indeed, Ecuadorian IVF patients and practitioners rarely took an absolutist stance towards any one model of causality in regards to moods and bodily state. The general acceptance of plurality on the part of patients also meshed well with a keen awareness by practitioners and patients of their own locatedness, their inability to assume a universal biology, and their acceptance of ambiguity, resonant with thinking in terms of what Margaret Lock calls "local biologies."[4]

When IVF practitioners spoke about their patients, and their bodily states, their comments were often couched in terms of comparison of their differences with others, both economic and physiological. These "local biologies" could be found in practitioners' comments about the administration of hormones and their effects upon local women.

IVF is a purposeful attempt to overstimulate a woman's ovaries to ripen more than one follicle. But the numbers of follicles or eggs produced through hormonal stimulation can also be classified as "excessive" and hyperstimulated. Ovarian hyperstimulation syndrome is probably the most common, negative, acute side effect of IVF. The hormonal stimulation of a woman's ovaries can overripen her follicles so they enlarge and cause abdominal cramping, excessive swelling, dehydration, which in some cases requires hospitalization. In Ecuador doctors routinely described how bodily states like hyperstimulation vary across national borders. One laboratory biologist, Diego explained that where he trained in Brazil the definition of hyperstimulation was sixty mature follicles. Back in Ecuador he called anything over twenty-five follicles hyperstimualtion, given that the average number of stimulated follicles was fifteen. He was clear that this average was determined by economics that affected physiology. Patients received a lower dosage of hormones in Ecuador because they had less money. Thus twenty-five follicles would represent a hyper-response to a lower dosage, while in Brazil sixty represented a hyper response to a much higher dose. By limiting their claims to the "local" practitioners, patients assumed the likelihood of plurality in interpreting bodily effects. Located bodies can differ from other bodies elsewhere. There is no *one* body or normative experience of embodiment. And located bodies can suffer from a *multiplicity* of afflictions that are not just the result of a *singular* agent.

In talking with physicians and patients I realized that they had already done the comparative work of thinking through what is particular to IVF in Ecuador. IVF was yet one more site in which to enact one's modernity, which also always entailed realizing one's biological and social distance from North America. Comparison to medicine in the US dominated the thinking of my research subjects as much, or more so, as it did my own. To be an urban mestizo Ecuadorian entails an acute sense of the decentered, of knowing oneself as local and specific, of never having the luxury of universalizing one's own experience. Those involved in IVF in Ecuador saw themselves as modern – but for them, modernity did not entail the universalism that characterizes modernity in Europe or North America (Trouillot 2002; Bauman 2001; Lock 1993).

Reproductive modernity

If biotechnologies like IVF are not wholly remaking Ecuadorians' understandings of biology or sociality as they are in the North, how have assisted reproductive technologies been received? Especially in marginalized nations one of the many pleasures bio-technologies offer is the participation in modernity, and the related set of distinctions this allows between oneself and the local, less-than-moderns, the poor, the backward, the indigenous. In Ecuador, women's reproductive failures are an expected part of the modern condition due to delayed childbearing, and the numerous "behavioral problems" of modern women. These failures required costly private fixes, which produced an identity as a moral consumer who is able to participate in the modern management of the failed female body. This is a biological and a social identity but not necessarily a biosocial one, as it does not fully entail a new relationship between the biological and the social as Rabinow describes for the United States and Europe.

In explaining infertility Ecuadorian IVF practitioners and patients narratized it as a "modern problem." This story is not limited to Ecuador by any means. Many of the factors that are thought to contribute to the "infertility epidemic" are the same for the United States and Europe, and are linked to ailments of modernity. A partial list of these problems must always begin with the "increase" of women in the work force which is presumed to lead to delayed childbearing. Other factors are thought to be pollution, occupational hazards, processed foods, the increase in premarital sex which leads to the rise in STDs, increased drug use and alcoholism, birth control methods like IUDs, and women's severe diet or exercise regime. Most of these factors presume a change in bodily comportment on the part of women who are modernizing.

In Ecuador, urban middle class women were primed to accept that their reproductive capacity is in disarray and measures should be taken to fix it, pills to swallow, drugs injections, surgeries undergone. Nowhere is this clearer than in the extreme rise in cesarean section in the last two decades. Cesarean sections are in part bodily signs of one's participation in a class based, private medical system. In private Ecuadorian clinics the c-section rate is 80–85 percent, while in urban publicly funded hospitals it is 22 percent, and rising. In rural areas it's about 8 percent. A sign of reproductive success for these women is giving birth at a private clinic which are numerous and advertised everywhere as opposed to giving birth vaginally, or suffering the horrors of the public maternity hospital. To be operated upon is a privilege of those who can afford to pay, and those who can pay are those who are most likely to have a malfunctioning body.

Most Ecuadorian women are well aware of the radical differences between public and private, urban and rural birth in terms of cesarean section. In addition the vast majority of middle class women I spoke with did not know a single woman of their generation who had a vaginal birth, or what is called " parto normal," or simply "lo normal," except their *empleadas* (domestic servants). For middle class Ecuadorian women calling vaginal birth "lo normal" is a clear declaration that their bodies deviate from the norm, since their bodies cannot support normal, vaginal birth. The normal in this case is the Indian, the rural *campesino*, the black woman and the poor urban woman, all who give birth in public hospitals or outside hospitals altogether. Linda, the laboratory biologist described above, told me that she was once allowed to watch a woman "attempt" to give birth vaginally at a private clinic (Linda had already had her children by c-section at that point). She was horrified and traumatized by the experience. For her it "was like watching torture." The woman screamed explosively and acted like "an animal, like a wild, savage woman." And in the end she had a cesarean section anyway. "What was the point?"

IVF babies were generally understood by both practitioners and patients as more precious, so were doubly fated for c-section birth, which was understood to minimize risk to these hard-won children. No doctor could imagine a woman giving birth vaginally after undergoing the expensive and chancy venture of IVF. One young IVF patient, Marta, who was a physician who worked in a public hospital, told me about how she had been thinking of having a "normal" birth for her IVF baby. But she was counseled by her mother to have c-section because she wouldn't be able to withstand the pain and ultimately was convinced by her IVF doctor to have a cesarean because of the particular preciousness of her IVF child.

> Dr. Jaramillo told me "you could give birth normally, if you want to give birth normally." Then my mother told me, "My daughter, to birth normally, is pain that you are not going to endure." Dr. Jaramillo told me "we could do the birth normally because the neck of your uterus is dilated, you are having contractions, but the truth," he told me "is that more pain is going to come." We could do a normal birth for you but I would not want to risk, what for you is, a very valuable product. We will do a cesarean for you." And I didn't think twice. I said to the doctor do the cesarean because in the first place my mother had gotten me alarmed about this question of pain, and second because it will happen quickly, the moment won't traumatize me. And I said, "do a cesarean doctor! Let's not wait any longer." When my little Isaac was born, everything was well. Thanks to God! You don't know the immense happiness when they took him out of me!

This woman's mild interest in attempting the "out of the ordinary feat" of having a "normal" birth was easily quelled through the warnings of her mother that she would be physically incapable of enduring the pain, and her doctor's concern about risking the "valuable product" that was Isaac. Although she had perhaps been more exposed to "normal" birth through her work in the hospital there was no support for this faint desire to attempt one. In Ecuador there was no culture of middle class vaginal birth to appeal to, no one to copy except for older women who imagine normal birth as lost to modernity, and for the better. Modern birth, meaning birth by cesarean section, is more secure and controlled, less animal, less savage. This control and safety is important for the bodies of modern women who cannot physically withstand labor.

Additionally, cesarean section secured the financial investment in the valuable product of an IVF baby, just as Dr. Jaramillo told Marta. The expense of IVF was of great consequence for the majority of IVF patients. But for many patients spending money to generate children was seen to have value in its own right. Their willingness to take on great debt and burden to alleviate their childlessness signified for them how much they wanted their children. Patients scraped together the money needed for IVF from their families, moneylenders and from small capital improvement loans they received for their businesses. Many couples would talk about doing IVF as an investment made, instead of buying a better house, bigger TV, or spending their money on some other big purchase. Carlos, a man with IVF twins explained: "It cost us a lot. We will tell them that they cost us a lot." His wife, Marisol agreed. "Yes they were very expensive. We had to work very hard to have them come." Another IVF patient, Laura, had not figured out how much money she had spent in total on IVF but told me that when she finally had a child she would tally up the total. Her first cycle did not work and she was contemplating a second.

> I have here the receipts. Sometimes we talk about the day that I have my child I will figure out how much it has all cost me. We have never done the accounts to see what we have spent. But it is money that it is not painful to see spent because, as we have said, we could have many more material things that would not compensate for what we are looking for in reality.

For Laura adding up accounts to figure out how much a child cost provided her with a way to equate a child with an amount of money. That price signaled the added financial sacrifice these parents made to have an IVF child beyond the usual sacrifices that any parent makes to raise offspring.

The need for caesareans, IVF and other reproductive treatments has become the norm for those with abnormal modern female bodies that require a modern fix. The embrace of IVF by urban middle class women in Ecuador demonstrates that these technologies reinforce and produce bodily identity as reproductively broken. In this way a dysfunctional uterus or childlessness is not only a stigma, but also is a sign of modernity, especially if one has the means to fix these problems with biomedical interventions. With cesarean scars, and IVF procedures, elite and middle class Ecuadorian women display themselves as reproductively modern, distinguishing their bodies from the functional bodies of poor, rural, black or Indian women. These normal women's bodies do not malfunction in the way that modern women's bodies do – whose menstruation is somehow always troublesome, who cannot withstand the pains of childbirth, and who cannot conceive. While IVF is now one among many reproductive procedures that shape the biological/social identity of modern women, it is not linked to new understanding of biology as malleable, or to collective social action around a biological identity. In Ecuador reproductive problems and the ability to consume for them are normal/pathological signs of modern consumption habits and modern physiology.

The normally pathological

The critical and ethnographic study of bioscience and technology outside cosmopolitan centers offers the potential to understand how "life" technologies are propagated and consumed within very different contexts, often in unanticipated ways. In Ecuador new technological practices have become a part of local conversations about modernity, sociality and biology that are different from those that have fostered biosociality in Europe and North America. In Ecuador both the biological and the social are important categories for experiencing the world but they *mean* differently. This divergent response serves to situate and povincialize biosociality as emanating from a specific time and place.

Ecuadorian women's flawed modern bodies do not necessarily function the same as the modern bodies of North American women. Even with the charisma of imported modern technologies, the modern bodies of Ecuadorian women partake in a fundamentally distinct epistemological approach to physiological causality than in the United States. Ecuadorian women undergoing hormonal IVF treatment experience their bodies as "local" instead of exemplars of universal biological processes. We might say then that North American and European biological understandings are becoming more like biology in the Andes, malleable and shaped by environmental factors, like education and class.

In *The Normal and the Pathological*, Georges Canguilhem described how:

> It is popularly said [that] … there is a difference between an organism and society, in that the therapist of their ills, in this case an organism, knows in advance and without hesitation what normal state to establish, while in the case of society he does not know.
>
> (Canguilhem 1991: 257)

Canguilhem countered this popular view of the biological fixity of the norm by mapping the shifting state of organic norms in medicine and science. In recent years these norms of biological fixity has begun to wane in North America and Europe while notions of biological plasticity and the need for the enhancement of the organism beyond health have become the new normal (Dumit 2002; Hogle 2005). These new forms of biological normality have similarities to current biological norms in Ecuador where modernity is a project that simultaneously produces biological dysfunction and fixes it. As Rabinow suggested, it is "worth monitoring" if this new norm of biological abnormality produce new biosocialites. In North American and European nations, where activist groups are doubtlessly already forming around these new norms, it might be. In Ecuador, other forms of embodied identity will most likely be produced through a different sociality and a different biology.

Acknowledgements

This article's development benefited greatly from the insightful comments and criticisms of Sahra Gibbon and Carlos Novas. I also want to thank them for organizing such a collegial and diverting workshop at the LSE in February 2006. The generous engagement of my fellow volume authors and participating scholars, at the workshop, was crucial in shaping the final draft. Additional thanks are due to Adi Bharadwaj, Nancy Scheper-Hughes, Lawrence Cohen, Lucinda Ramberg and Gay Becker for their help in conceptualizing my initial thoughts about reproductive modernity in Ecuador. The Wenner Gren and the National

Science Foundation provided generous funding for the bulk of my Ecuadorian research.

Notes

1 The research for this chapter is based on an ongoing engagement with Ecuadorian IVF since 2000. In 2002–3, I carried out a year of ethnographic research in seven of Ecuador's nine private IVF clinics. My observations mainly took place in the IVF clinics themselves, watching and talking with practitioners and patients in waiting rooms, laboratories, operating rooms, and patients' recovery rooms. In addition I conducted over 130 formal interviews for the project with: female infertility patients, their male partners, IVF practitioners, physicians, laboratory biologists, and staff at IVF clinics, egg and sperm donors, surrogate mothers, local Catholic priests, lawyers and bio-ethicists. For an expanded discussion of my findings see my dissertation "Equatorial *In-Vitro*: Reproductive Medicine and Modernity in Ecuador" (2006, U.C. Berkeley).
2 IVF clinics serve a predominantly middle to upper income clientele with monthly salaries ranging from $800 to $2,000. IVF cycles in Ecuador cost from $4,500–$6,000.
3 For additional examples of biosociality defined primarily through groupings and identities see Dumit 2004; Franklin and Lock 2003; Petryna 2002; Biehl 2005.
4 In her book *Encounters With Aging* Margaret Lock (1993) introduced the concept of "local biologies" to describe the complex interplay of history, political economy, and society that formulates the physiological iteration of bodies in specific local times and places. Local biologies undo the notion that "biology is immutable" while culture is malleable (p. 373). In Lock's formulation the situatedness of biological experiences is "not simply the result of culturally shaped interpretations of a universal physical experience but the products ... of an ongoing dialectic between biology and culture in which both are contingent" (p. xxi).

References

Bauman, Zygmunt (2001) Modernity. In *The Bauman Reader*. P. Beilharz, ed. pp. xi, 365. Blackwell Readers. Malden, MA: Blackwell Publishers.

Becker, Gay (2000) *The Elusive Embryo. How Women and Men Approach New Reproductive Technologies*. Berkeley, CA: University of California Press.

Biehl, João Guilherme (2005) *Vita: Life in a Zone of Social Abandonment*. Berkeley, CA: University of California Press.

Bustamante, Marco (1989) "Bebes Probeta" 100% Ecuatorianos: Los Niños del Millón de Sucres. *Vistazo*: 39–42.

Cadena, Marisol de la (2000) *Indigenous Mestizos: The Politics of Race and Culture in Cuzco, 1919–1991*. Durham, NC: Duke University Press.

Canguilhem, Georges (1991) *The Normal and the Pathological*. New York: Zone Books.

CEPAR (2000) *Endemain-III, Ecuador Informe General*. Quito: Centro de Estudios de Poblacion y Desarrollo Social.

Colloredo-Mansfeld, Rudi (1998) "Dirty Indians," Radical Indigenas and the Political Economy of Social Difference in Modern Ecuador. *Bulletin of Latin American Research*, 17(2): 185–205.

Das, Veena (2001) Stigma, Contagion, Defect: Issues in the Anthropology of Public Health. Stigma and Global Health Conference. Bethesda, Maryland, 2001.

Davis, Dona Lee, and Setha M. Low (1989) *Gender, Health, and Illness: The Case of Nerves.* New York: Hemisphere.

Dumit, Joseph (2002) Drugs for Life. *Molecular Interventions*, 2(3): 124–7.

Dumit, Joseph (2004) *Picturing Personhood: Brain Scans and Biomedical Identity.* Princeton, NJ: Princeton University Press.

Foucault, Michel (1990) *The History of Sexuality.* New York: Vintage Books.

Franklin, Sarah and Margaret M. Lock (2003) *Remaking Life and Death: Toward an Anthropology of the Biosciences.* Santa Fe and Oxford: School of American Research Press.

Gerlach, Allen (2003) *Indians, Oil, and Politics: A Recent History of Ecuador.* Wilmington, DE: Scholarly Resources.

Gomez, Sara (1991) El Bebé Probeta Llego a Ecuador: Los Hijos de la Ciencia. *La Otra*: 62–5.

Gordon, Deborah (1988) Tenacious Assumptions in Western Medicine. In M. M. Lock and D. R. Gordon (eds) *Biomedicine Examined: Culture, Illness, and Healing.* Dordrecht and Boston, MA: Kluwer Academic Publishers.

Hogle, Linda (2005) Enhancement Technologies and the Body. *Annual Review of Anthropology*, 34: 695–716.

Keller, Evelyn Fox (2000) *The Century of the Gene.* Cambridge, MA: Harvard University Press.

Krupa, Christopher (2005) *State by Proxy: Race Politics, Labor, and the Shifting Morphology of Governance in Highland Ecuador.* Dissertation. University of California, Davis

Lock, Margaret M. (1993) *Encounters with Aging: Mythologies of Menopause in Japan and North America.* Berkeley, CA: University of California Press.

Lock, Margaret M. and Deborah Gordon (1988) *Biomedicine Examined.* Dordrecht and Boston, MA: Kluwer Academic Publishers.

Mallon, Florencia (1996) Constructing Mestizaje in Latin America: Authenticity, Marginality, and Gender in the Claiming of Ethnic Identities. *Journal of Latin American Anthropology*, 2(1): 170–81.

Orlove, Benjamin (1998) Down to Earth: Race and Substance in the Andes. *Bulletin of Latin American Research*, 17(2): 207–22.

Oudshoorn, Nelly (1994) *Beyond the Natural Body: An Archaeology of Sex Hormones.* New York and London: Routledge.

Petryna, Adriana (2002) *Life Exposed: Biological Citizens after Chernobyl.* Princeton, NJ: Princeton University Press.

Poole, Deborah (1997) *Vision, Race, and Modernity: A Visual Economy of the Andean Image World.* Princeton, NJ: Princeton University Press.

Poole, Deborah (2004) Between Threat and Guarantee: Justice and Community in the Margins of the Peruvian State. In V. Das and D. Poole (eds) *Anthropology in the Margins of the State.* Santa Fe, NM: School of American Research Press.

Rabinow, Paul (1996) Artificiality and Enlightenment: From Sociobiology to Biosociality. In *Essays on the Anthropology of Reason.* Princeton, NJ: Princeton University Press.

Rapp, Rayna (1999) *Testing Women, Testing the Fetus: The Social Impact of Amniocentesis in America.* New York: Routledge.

Roberts, Elizabeth (1998a) Examining Surrogacy Discourses: Between Feminine Power and Exploitation. In N. Scheper-Hughes and C. Sargent (eds) *Small Wars: The Cultural Politics of Childhood.* Berkeley, CA: University of California Press.

Roberts, Elizabeth (1998b) "Native" Narratives of Connectedness Surrogate Motherhood and Technology. In J. Dumit and R. Davis-Floyd (eds) *Cyborg Babies: From Techno-Sex to Techno-Tots.* New York: Routledge.

Rose, Nikolas, and Carlos Novas (2005) Biological Citizenship. In A. Ong and S. J. Collier (eds) *Global Assemblages: Technology, Politics, and ethics as Anthropological Problems*. Malden, MA: Blackwell Publishing.

Scheper-Hughes, Nancy (1992) *Death Without Weeping: The Violence of Everyday Life in Brazil*. Berkeley, CA: University of California Press.

Sommers, Doris (2002) Love and Country: An Allegorical Speculation from Foundational Fictions: The National Romances of Latin America. In B. Trigo (ed.) *Foucault and Latin America: Appropriations and Deployments of Discursive Analysis*. New York: Routledge.

Leyes Stepan, Nancy (1982) *The Idea of Race in Science: Great Britain, 1800–1960*. London: Macmillan in association with St Antony's College Oxford.

Leyes Stepan, Nancy (1991) *The Hour of Eugenics: Race, Gender, and Nation in Latin America*. Ithaca, NY: Cornell University Press.

Stoler, Ann Laura (1995) *Race and the Education of Desire: Foucault's History of Sexuality and the Colonial Order of Things*. Durham, NC: Duke University Press.

Strathern, Marilyn (1992) *After Nature: English Kinship in the Late Twentieth Century*. Cambridge and New York: Cambridge University Press.

Stutzman, Ronald (1981) El Mestizaje. An All Inclusive Ideology. In N. Whitten (ed.) *Cultural Transformations and Ethnicity in Modern Ecuador*. Urbana, IL: University of Illinois.

Trouillot, Michel-Rolph (2002) The Otherwise Modern. Caribbean Lessons from the Savage Slot. In B. M. Knauft (ed.) *Critically Modern Alternatives, Alterities, Anthropologies*. Bloomington, IN: Indiana University Press.

Vos, Rob, José Cuesta, Mauricio León, Ruth Lucio, and José Rosero (2004) *Ecuador, Public Expenditure Review 2004, Health*. Quito: Secretaria Tecnica del Frente Social.

Wade, Peter (1993) Race, Nature and Culture. *Man*, 28(1): 17–34.

Weismantel, Mary J. (2001) *Cholas and Pishtacos: Stories of Race and Sex in the Andes*. Chicago, IL: University of Chicago Press.

Whitten, Norman E. (2003) *Millennial Ecuador: Critical Essays on Cultural Transformations and Social Dynamics*. Iowa City, IA: University of Iowa Press.

World Health Organization (WHO) (2005) Statistics by Country or Region, Ecuador.

5 Biosociality and biocrossings

Encounters with assisted conception and embryonic stem cells in India

Aditya Bharadwaj

Introduction

The anthropological imagination has variously conceptualised the constructed nature of the biological, organic, natural and their shifting meanings. Alongside biosociality (Rabinow, 1992) conceptual incisions like the hybrids (Latour, 1993), juxtapositions (Strathern, 1992) and cyborgs (Haraway, 1990, 1991) have similarly problematised the post/late modern *bioscapes*. That is, a terrain of analysis examining the fundamental rupture, implosion of the social and that which was conceptualised as the domain of the natural in the post-Enlightened Euro-America. These insights have on the one hand enriched the social sciences conceptually and methodologically but on the other privileged the existence of one among many other possible cultural biographies of human biology. The very act of demolishing the hegemonic formulations of nature/culture oppositions in the Euro-American worldview has unwittingly led to the 'anthropologisation' of an equally dominant model of the biological and the social that continually bleed into each other. When globalised such conceptual tropes present hitherto unexamined complexities.[1] For example, the 'biological' encountered in Indian *in vitro* fertilisation (IVF) and stem cell laboratories is often an amalgam of multiple 'indigenous' notions of the body and bio-scientific models of human biology (invoked by clinicians and scientists trained in 'Western and Indian' academies). This is in distinction to a vulgar nature/culture split or a more nuanced nature/culture implosion. In other words, while nature is being produced and remade as culture in the 'local moral worlds' of anthropologists, such conceptualisations have little purchase in the globally dispersed lives of scientists and 'patients' whose bodies become points of technological application. I have observed in various IVF and stem cell research laboratories, for instance, how 'patients' and clinicians/scientists alike tend not to view critically the implosions of nature and culture. Instead they continually appropriate the supposed difference into familiar categories (such as kinship and relatedness). Thus for the anthropologist this is something new in the making, i.e. kinship, family, parenthood is itself being remade by fracturing older conceptualisations.[2] In contrast, in the everyday lived experience of the 'Indian infertile patients' this is yet another instance of improvisation in their efforts to re-establish the normative and the ideologically compliant. The secrecy surrounding donor gamete conception in Indian IVF has led me to conclude that 'kinship authorises just as it authors the process of conception' (Bharadwaj, 2003). That is, by subsuming the process of donor assisted conception in silence, individuals and couples are able to craft normatively unproblematic kinship. Assisted conception can create separate and new categories such as social, genetic, gestational or biological parents and kin (Strathern, 1992: 20). In the Indian context, however, it is not seen as instantiating the 'new' but rather facilitating and enabling the 'familiar' i.e. socially visible parenthood where biological is misrecognised in favour of social relations (Bharadwaj, 2003).

Against this backdrop how might the notion of biosociality explain local and global cultural complexities underlying the experience of health and illness? As a concept does it successfully capture the unprecedented rise and spread of new biotechnologies around the globe? In other words, whilst the concept has significantly altered social science engagements with emergent complexities underscoring 'biological life' it can, nevertheless, be challenged to explain and contain a lot more in a world suffused with bewildering cultural and biotechnological disparity.

In this chapter, therefore, I will examine the concept of biosociality in its present shape and form and propose limitations that emerge when it is applied to a rapidly transforming India. In so doing, I (re)conceptualise the *bio* as *available* as opposed to *social* by focusing on the processes of extraction and insertion that not only generate 'biovalue', but also facilitate what I will call *biocrossings*. To argue this point further I open two tentative ethnographic registers describing the clinical application of biotechnologies of assisted conception and embryonic stem cells in India.

Biosociality: the excluded 'others'?

> In the future, the new genetics will cease to be a biological metaphor for modern society and will become instead a circulation network of identity terms and restriction loci, around which and through which a truly new type of autoproduction will emerge, which I call biosociality.
>
> (Rabinow, 1996: 98)

It is perhaps fair to say that the notion of biosociality was never intended to be a 'master concept' seeking to unpack conundrums and complexities associated with the human biological form and its social context around the globe. It is not simply the case that the notion of biosociality is inadequate and that we must now expand the formulation to include the 'excluded others' but rather what is important is the predictive voice in which the concept was first enunciated almost fifteen years ago. Many of the predictions have stood the test of time (cf. Rapp, 2000) and some others await fruition. Two of the most important pronouncements about the future encapsulated in the idea of biosociality are well known:

1   In the future ... likely formation of new groups and individual identities
    and practices arising out of [these] new truths ...
2   ... nature will be made known and remade through technique and will
    finally become artificial, just as culture becomes natural ...

(Rabinow, 1996: 99–102)

It is difficult to conjure a temporal dimension. To engage with the future is
to imagine it, just as to engage with the past is to reinvent it. In both cases the
processes at work are that of prediction and remembrance. However if time can
be remembered and predicted, then clearly the present can only be actualised
in experience. The futures predicted when the concept was first proposed have
potential to be actualised and experienced in contexts that are not universally
available. Therefore, for the concept of biosociality to be viable its cultural and
temporal contours must be outlined. Rabinow takes the American Human Genome
Initiative (AHGI) as one 'logical place to begin' an examination of changes to
life in the context of new knowledge and power. If anything, the contours of his
project are precisely drawn and defined. In this respect his ethnographic question
is clear, he asks: How will our social and ethical practices change as this project
(AHGI) advances? The very idea of 'our social and ethical practices' is posited
at the notable expense of excluding those who seemingly do not fit the Euro-
American category.[3] I do not make this observation as a critique but rather to
further emphasise the point that the idea of biosociality is limited in the global
context and this is because perhaps as a concept it was never intended to travel
very far in the first place.

In global spaces, like India, biotechnologies are available and thriving as
opposed to locales both within India and elsewhere where crippling poverty
asphyxiates, often prematurely, both the 'bio' and any semblance of 'sociality'.
Such ethnographic 'truths' cannot be wished away if anthropology is to continue
to understand, explain and critique the 'difference' that permeates the world. The
conceptual and anthropological challenge therefore is to remain in an anticipatory
space, one that does not seek to pre-empt 'difference' through intuitively second-
guessing its emergence but rather by being alert to its possible existence. In this
respect this essay can be read on two levels: as a problematisation of the concept
of biosociality and as a first tentative step towards further elaborating the concept
through critical thinking. Whilst I personally prefer the latter reading, different
readers will no doubt bring different interpretations. It is the act of reading, and
not necessarily writing that eventually creates a text.

My research concerns in India thus far can be distilled and framed as follows:
how do people seeking biomedical interventions persist in an emerging neoliberal
formation like India on terms far out of their control, certainly not of their choosing
and seldom of their own making? The same question can be posed elsewhere.
However the question and the terrain it instantiates seems appropriate for an
analysis that seeks to bring into focus biosociality of individuals and potential
groupings who find the lived experience of their bodies irreversibly scarred
by the neoliberal statecraft and political economy. And yet the complexities

and compulsions individuals and/or collectivities face in emerging neoliberal formations like India (Bharadwaj, 2006c) seldom produce powerful opportunities to harness or gain anything remotely profitable from being biosocially active. The constraints are multiple from unavailability of opportunity, resources and ability to organise around a medical condition, syndrome, mutation to the social isolation, stigma and delegitimation. I will further explore these themes in my ethnographic illustrations.

Biocrossing, extraction, insertion

Whilst a lot of ink has been spilt on the neoliberal agenda around the globe I find Paul Farmer's (2003) formulation most lucid and helpful to contextualise neoIndia. Describing the competition driven market model of neoliberalism Farmer argues how within this doctrine:

> [...] individuals in a society are viewed, if viewed at all, as autonomous, rational producers and consumers whose decisions are motivated primarily by economic or material concerns. But this ideology has little to say about the social and economic inequalities that distort real economies.
>
> (Farmer, 2003: 5)

The distorted face of neoliberal economies is further exacerbated if we add to the picture the parallel bioeconomies and, following Waldby (2002), the promissory biovalue they hope to generate. According to Catherine Waldby:

> Biovalue refers to the yield of vitality produced by the biotechnological reformulation of living processes. Biotechnology tries to gain traction in living processes. To induce them to increase or change their productivity along specified lines, intensify their self-reproducing and self-maintaining capacities. This intensification or leveraging of living process typically takes place not at the level of the body as a macro-anatomical system but at the level of the cellular or molecular fragment, the mRNA, the bacterium, the oocyte, the stem cell.
>
> (Waldby, 2002: 310)

Such a way of capitalising on life according to Walby produces a margin of biovalue, a surplus of fragmentary vitality. There are two incentives according to her in the production of biovalue: First, *the public incentive* or the biosociality of advocates (though Walby doesn't use the concept) hoping for the creation of a *use value*. A good example is the promissory future emerging from stem cell therapies. Second, the incentive is to generate *exchange value*, biological commodities that can be bought and sold in a purportedly 'free market'. However, whereas in capitalism, capital is accumulated, in biomedical enterprise, capital is promissory (Thompson, 2005) that is capital raised for speculative ventures on the strength of promised future returns (Franklin, 2003).

Waldby's thesis rightly identifies generation of biovalue through intensification of living processes at the molecular level or other levels of similar scale that require microscopic gaze as opposed to macro-anatomical systems. However, the very act of generating biovalue makes the macro-anatomical system valuable in the market driven neoliberal mode of production. This value is achieved through the twin processes of *extraction* and *insertion*. The process of *extraction* makes the macro-anatomical a priceless site for harvesting raw biomaterials and as a site for *insertion* a locale for witnessing the promised *use value* itself. Whilst the former is most graphically literalised in public and academic debates surrounding the use of embryos for stem cell research or the harvesting of human organs for transplants the latter is yet to capture the world's imagination. For example, as yet there are no scientifically documented instances of embryonic stem cell *insertions* in macro-anatomical systems. I will however later show how *extraction* and *insertion* of embryonic stem cells is being accomplished and the resultant question of biovalue is being addressed in India. The importance and centrality of the macro-anatomical in micro biotech interventions is therefore indispensable and another good reason to resist Donna Haraway's (1990) clarion call to write the death of the clinic (Bharadwaj *et al.*, 2006a).

The generation of biovalue through the process of extraction and insertion on the other hand is enabled because macro-anatomical sites become bioavailable in the first place. Lawrence Cohen's (2004, 2005) lucid formulation captures the very process whereby selective disaggregation of one's cells or tissues and their reincorporation into another body is made possible. In addition to Lawrence's evocative usage bioavailability in the realm of medicine is taken to mean the degree to which a drug or *other substance* can be absorbed and utilised by those parts of the body on which it is intended to have an effect. That is, the proportion of a drug which reaches its site of pharmacological activity when introduced into the body (*Oxford Concise*, 2006, emphasis added). Taken together these two different meanings of bioavailability bring into focus topographies of bioavailable transfers of cellular and tissue based entities mediated by technical and biological processes that either facilitate or stifle the absorption/utilization by those parts of the body on which such transferred biogenetic entities are intended to have an effect. These transfers – achieved through extraction and insertion and administered as an intended medical resolution of a pre-existing social or medical problem – I will term *biocrossing*. This is a crossing between biology, biology and machine and across geo-political, commercial, ethical and moral borders. 'Bio' on the other hand can be visualised as an ethnoscientific rendition of the 'human biological' and as such stands – not necessarily opposed to – multiple crosscultural conceptualisations of human biology. Thus bio can be gainfully conceptualised as an instance of *biologically based biography*, be it individual (e.g. an illness narrative or cultural/'ethno' conception of human body) or institutional (bio-science/medicine/technology etc.). A biography is inextricably inserted in any individual and/or institutional understanding of the biological.[4] The anthropological and ethnographic endeavour in this respect is to decode the biographical inscriptions that produce, sustain and alter the bio through multiple crossings across various borders and thresholds. This makes bio a site in which the discipline of anthropology, science, bioavailable 'patients' and subaltern subjectivities are all equally implicated. Biocrossing in this respect is crossings made in a contested terrain, in which anthropological assertions about imploding boundaries between nature, culture, biology, society need to be problematised alongside the scientific dogma and everyday negotiating practices of those who find their bodies double up as sites for both an enactment of new scientific applications and their anthropological narration. Bio therefore can never have a stable conceptual mooring not because it is continually remade but rather 'crossed over' between assemblages of different cultural terrains (cf. Ong and Collier, 2005). The notion of an assemblage when invoked as dispersed in the Marxist usage purports to an idea of use value that may be looked at from the point of view of 'quantity' and 'quality' of any useful 'thing' (in the Marxist formulation these were things like iron, paper, etc. though in the present case substituted by the idea of the [bio]logical). Thus 'it' (useful thing) is an:

> *assemblage of many properties*, and may therefore be of *use* in various ways [extraction, insertion etc]. To discover the various uses of things [such as the very idea of bio and its use value] is the work of history. So also is the establishment of socially-recognised standards of measure [e.g. bio-medicine/technology] for the quantities [such as bodies and bodily tissues] of these useful objects. The diversity of these measures has its origin partly in the *diverse nature of the objects* [e.g. Nature of an object will amount to its discursive contours such as bio, body, 'ethno' physiology] to be measured, partly in *convention*.
>
> (Marx, 1963: 43, emphasis added)

Thus an assemblage has both historic depth and future potential; it actualises the past and futures into the present not so much through severing all connections from temporality but by incorporating such links into the shifting use value of a given 'thing' by (re)measuring it in the present using the 'conventional' or normative standard of the day. That this value is produced through a multitude of 'qualities' and 'quantities' is the single most important signifier of an assemblage. Biocrossing therefore amounts to a contextual, contingent and temporal movement of the human body (itself a cultural, historic and political assemblage) across tangible, material, philosophical, historical, political, and many more 'fictional' borders of varying scale.

When I describe 'actors' in Indian IVF and stem cell clinics and laboratories as bioavailable and not biosocial I am essentially drawing on biocrossing emerging from two different readings of the term bioavailable. The individuals in Indian IVF and stem cell clinics emerge not only as bioavailable in that they can be used for extraction and insertion for generating biovalue, but also because the ways in which their failing biology absorbs, processes, rejects, or accepts – hormones, sperm, eggs, embryos, stem cells – is highly unpredictable. In a word while they are bioavailable to science (predicated on the rhetoric of pre-treatment counselling, informed consent and choice) for generating exchange and use value, what is bioavailable to their biology in terms of actual tangible benefits is highly variable.

Reproductive disruptions: biocrossing the 'barren' terrain

On the morning of 5th April 1997 two men accompanied with their wives accosted me right outside the clinic. I had spotted them in deep animated conversation from quite some distance as I was approaching the clinic. On closer inspection I recognised one of the two couples – Sumita and Shankar – as I had interviewed them a day before. Shankar took me to a side looking visibly upset and asked me in a low, hushed secretive tone if I could come to his hotel room sometime later in the day as he wanted to tell me something about the doctor. At this point the other man joined us and shouted how there is no humanity in the country. 'The doctor here is after money, money and more money, there is no humanity, show some humanity at least' he sneered. I was beginning to get confused not knowing what fresh event(s) brought on this diatribe against the doctor. Even as I was pondering over the possible reasons – either the treatment wasn't progressing to their liking or the expenses involved were beyond their means – the man retorted to my confused silence 'look at the national culture of money making, look at our Prime Minster, can anything go right in a country whose leader is so incompetent'. At this point Shankar chipped in 'there is no humanity and no nationality [sic I think what he meant was a feeling of nationalism] in the country, the doctors are interested only in your money!' Later in the day I went around to their hotel to find out what was on Shankar and Sumita's minds. 'The doctor doesn't give us a clear estimate ever on how much it is all going to cost' they griped. At first instance the grouse seemed a bit of a damp-squib in relation to the morning's outburst but a subsequent chat with the couple revealed how when viewed in the context of their daily struggles one could make better sense of the emotional roller coaster they were straddling for the past 16 years. They have been coming to this clinic since 24.10.96 and maintain that they don't have to this day a realistic estimate of how much the whole treatment will amount to. Especially given that they travel an enormous distance to the clinic it is not possible or even financially viable for them to make trips to and fro to get more money, which they mobilise in their hometown of Dungarpur on the Northwestern tip of Gujarat State. While they acknowledged that the doctor was accommodating to the point of letting them pay the balance due, in an event of them running short of money, on their subsequent visits they were deeply upset with the person responsible for collections. Clearly the communication gap between the doctor and the staff was the cause of undue harassment. In the morning on requesting to pay the balance on their next visit the cashier reportedly said something 'obnoxious and rude' that triggered the emotional outburst outside the clinic. Paying for an expensive medical intervention they could ill afford was in their case mainly a function of conforming to social expectations and definitions of socially responsible behaviour. Shankar was hit by a personal tragedy earlier in 1996 when he lost his father. They had to rush back home abandoning the treatment mid way. Continuing to explain his present financial struggle he spoke of how meeting the expenses of his father's last rites added to his financial worries. 'The society expects it' he ruefully added while emphasising that any compromises or economising in the proper discharge of the last rites invites social disapproval and ridicule. He likened this to society not approving of individuals who don't make all out effort to secure a child should natural conception fail. Both husband and wife believed that social change is law of nature suggesting that 'everything in nature (Prakriti) changes including the customs, traditions, attitudes but to stand up against the contemporary norms is impossible, you have to conform'.

(Bharadwaj, 2001)[5]

The couple had pulled numerous threads from their biography that framed their struggle to become biological parents and their long-drawn financial drain. The impromptu invocation of the materialistic national culture and the incompetence of the prime minister by the man in the morning resonated with the couple as bearing testimony to the money-grabbing and impersonal inclinations of clinical medicine. Though they were reasonably happy with the way the doctor accommodated their requests to pay the balance on their subsequent visits to the clinic, they nevertheless held him responsible for the inhuman attitude of his staff. In doing this they drew parallels between widespread desire for material gain and the political culture that sustains it, seeing the commercialisation of clinical medicine as but one feature reflecting in microcosm the state of the nation. Shankar had conjured a tangled web of complex ideas that he later summed up in an ancient Sanskrit proverb that alludes to subjects reflecting the virtues of the king (*yatha raja taha praja*). The couple highlighted how the need to conform to socially defined expectations in respect of birth and death was making it obligatory for them to go beyond their means. They were trapped in an isolating silence and making themselves bioavailable to any medical intervention offered to salvage their fertility. Both Sumita and Shankar were grappling with secondary infertility since the death of their only child – a daughter – in 1976.

SHANKAR: 1981 the treatment started. We went to Ahemdabad and lots of other places, we went to a lot of places in Gujarat. They gave us hormonal treatment but no result. Nothing came of it!

AB: What do the doctors have to say about your case?

SHANKAR: A lot of doctors used to say 'you don't make ova' while the other lot said that the cycles are not proper.

AB: What kind of treatment was prescribed?

SHANKAR: All were hormonal treatments.

AB: Did you experience any side affects?

SHANKAR: Yes! She put on a lot of weight, cysts in the ovaries [interrupted]

SUMITA: Twice I had cysts in the ovaries!
AB: Any other complications?
SHANKAR: More cysts all because of these hormones!

For over 16 years, Sumita's body was at the receiving end of hormonal therapy, inflicted on her by the very doctors that she and Shankar turned to for help. At the time of these interviews and interactions both time and money was running out for them. Their biocrossing was in a terrain fraught with dangerous hormonal treatments, donor eggs, commuting great distance from home to seek treatment, raising money on interest and enduring overbearing social expectations that demanded both the beginning and the end of life be socially witnessed. The multiple thresholds they crossed, sometimes on a daily basis, entwined their unyielding reproductive biology and biography.

Social pressure to conceive is often crippling and it is not just the desperate poor, or financially weak couples that bear the brunt. A clinician in Delhi narrates a middle class encounter:

> [...] you will be surprised that a few days back I had a lady walk in with her daughter-in-law and I am telling you, I mean this will tell you the kind of pressures that there are; a young girl, so she said [referring to the mother-in-law] 'Oh! you know every month she starts menstruating', I was really taken aback by the crude way it was put. 'What's the problem, she is not conceiving?' I said 'how long has she been married?' that's the first question in a history that you would ask and I'll give you a guess, what do you think it was? Just take a guess! Four months! FOUR MONTHS!! Can you imagine the kind of pressure; just imagine the kind of pressure the poor kid was under, her mother-in-law is watching every menstrual cycle! This is pathetic, that's the kind of social pressure there is in the country ...
>
> (Bharadwaj, 2001)

The severity of pressure from family not surprisingly adds to the urgency with which married couples turn to clinical medicine for help. Thus another clinician in Mumbai argues that:

> The social pressure to have your own child is much, much higher in India. The social pressure is more within a year of marriage. People start telling the wife or the daughter-in-law 'why are you not conceiving? Why don't you see this doctor? See that doctor! Go to this temple, go here, go there' you know it starts within a year of marriage ... plus there is a lot of social pressure from friends, relatives, everyone [is asking] why are you not conceiving? So they [the couple] seek treatment very early. You will be surprised that 19 year old if she doesn't conceive by a year, by 20 she comes for treatment! Even if we say we will go slow, we don't want to do laparoscopy these are operative things we will do them after two years or so [as a last resort], nothing doing

they walk into the clinic next door. That's the kind of pressure they are under, they want instant results, they want fast treatment.

(Bharadwaj, 2001)

Stigmatised bodies that become bioavailable for hormonal treatments and biological materials like eggs, sperm and embryos often undertake biocrossing to manage their socially assigned identities of 'barren inauspiciousness' (Inhorn and Bharadwaj, 2007). Constrained by the overweening pro-natalist patriarchal expectations the only sociality women are able to exercise is to cooperate with the discipline of clinical medicine and that of the wider joint familial network with a vested interest in their reproductive biology. In crossing this terrain women, as in the examples above, negotiate the anomalous space where biography inscribes biology and biology frames the altering face of biography. The following entry in the journal – made on 4 June 1998 – gives an insight into how 'bio' and the 'social' are crossed in clinical encounters.

A young couple enters the room.

DR: You have a lovely wife!

M: Thank you!

DR: [addressing the woman] How old are you?

W: 24 years old, married for two years.

DR: Do you work?

W: No. I am a housewife. No intentions of working.

DR: [joking] Lucky! [...]

After a detailed case history the doctor asks the couple how she can help.

M: I only want a baby. I am prepared for everything. I am living in a joint family, my younger brother got married last year and his wife is pregnant. I live in a joint family and find it very difficult ... I'll do anything [alluding to a sperm test].

DR: [addressing his wife] You are 24, there is a lot of time [...]

The doctor sensing the anxiety in the couple began by explaining the impact of stress on the endocrinal system.

DR: The hypothalamus orders the pituitary to begin its work. FSH and LH [hormones secreted by the pituitary gland] come down to the ovaries where eggs are already present and the FSH and LH stimulate the ovaries and the eggs are matured.

Continuing, she explains the entire process again, this time using an analogy to make it more accessible:

DR: ... if the elders in the family are not good what will the junior or younger people do in such a family? If the family elders set a bad example for the younger lot, what can be expected of the young ones? Look at our country, if our political system is so bad what will become of the country? Same way, the hypothalamus has to set the right example for the pituitary in order for it to be able to stimulate the ovaries. So keep tensions away as it affects the proper functioning of the hypothalamus.

Please promise me you will leave all your troubles here with me. I had a patient who used to call me at 8 o'clock in the evening saying 'my mother-in-law is scolding me' [interrupted]

M: This way she will call you ten, fifteen times a day [laughs].

DR: [smiles and continues] I told her that either take your husband and go out or if he is scared of his mother you cook for her and pray. She is so pretty just like you and she is so tense. Please promise me that you will not think about these tensions anymore.

The clinician outlines how biographies of individuals can be inextricably liked to their biology and biological outcomes. She drives home the biomedical visualisation of the division of labour in the working of the endocrinal system by marrying it to the delicate power balance in the couple's joint family. The clinician invokes the metaphor of hierarchical familial relations and the rights and obligations that go with such relations. The analogy of a family patriarch setting the right example for the 'juniors' to follow, in the context of counselling, doubles up as an oblique reference to the couple's predicament – which is loaded with undue family pressure to conceive – as irresponsibility on the part of the elders of the (joint) family in allowing the burden to conceive to add to the couple's stress. Sensing anxiety in the man, the doctor appears to deliberately take up the example of one of her other patients, obliquely alluding to the importance of a husband supporting his wife, in the face of hostility from the mother-in-law, by suggesting that a woman who is unable to enlist her husband's support can do little other than cook to please her in-laws or pray. The doctor in other words addresses one of the core biographical subtexts underpinning the cause of stress in the couple's life by splicing it with explanations that seek to explain how biographies impact biology. She does this surreptitiously – by urging the couple to leave all their troubles with her, thus encouraging them to tackle the source of stress in their lives – for openly 'biocrossing' these sensitive issues may be viewed as lying outside of her professional remit.

Biocrossing 'emerging life forms': embryonic stem cell insertions

Through the course of my residence in Geeta Shroff's stem cell research laboratory and clinic in New Delhi in 2004–5, I encountered nearly 20 'patients' responding to embryonic stem cell trials for conditions as diverse as post-stroke to heart conditions such as sick sinus syndrome and left ventricular ejection fraction to cases of spinal damage and paralysis. In the global age of stem cells alongside the real danger of human exploitation emerges the real tantalising potential for cures. In several cases I found patients from all over India and as far away as Britain and the United State biocrossing to New Delhi to try stem cells as the medicine of last resort, their only hope. These individuals and their accompanying family members I recently argued have begun to acquire 'biological citizenship' in that they exist in the 'political economy of hope' (Rose and Novas, 2005: 442) and whilst their bio-sociality (Rabinow, 1996) is as yet not fully expressed and faced with life threatening conditions they remain unable to articulate the 'doubled discourse' of acceptance and normalisation (Rapp, 2000) they will perhaps one day get biosocially organised (Bharadwaj, 2006a).

I had made this hopeful statement at the time not reflecting enough on the biological biographies that shape their everyday struggles. In all my encounters ranging from infertility to the complex and diverse pool of degenerative diseases seeking embryonic stem cells as medicine I found actors focused on the question of resolution, relief, redemption, rescue, restitution rather than biosocial mobilisation. They have a vested investment in the therapies that Dr Shroff can offer, in many cases with dramatic breakthroughs and outcomes. They are nevertheless not assembling around their failing biology with the view to actively carving out a sociality. Their biological and social bodies are simply too frail, isolated and stigmatised to accomplish this.

Curious to understand what motivates women to make their infertile bodies and spare embryos bioavailable for stem cell extraction, I conducted 40 interviews. The resounding message that emerged was one of heart-breaking indifference that can only be described as 'indifferent altruism' and paraphrased to read: 'perhaps my ravaged body can rescue someone else's decaying, dying body'. The most disturbing moment was encountered when I sat speaking to a scared, visibly distraught woman in her early thirties who stared manically into the distance and simply responded to my compassionately worded question with 'spare embryos, sure, you can have my kidneys if you like, just get me pregnant'. The person in question was from a middle class family and like many women I have spoken to over the years was embracing a 'fertile' biotechnology to save her collapsing marriage and ward off the threat of abandonment. The space that distraught hapless and helpless women like her occupy also is a space that eventually becomes marked for bio-extraction. The spare IVF embryos, a curious entity that has come into existence ever since the science of embryonic transfers and stem cell became thinkable/doable, begin their long circuitous journey in these marked spaces. Most embryos, however, end up in research facilities dotted across the country doing no more than routine 'normal science'. They do however create clean paper trails of informed consent and free will that mark the embryos themselves as ethically unproblematic and neutral, masking the social suffering that lies hidden beneath yards of consent forms.

Dr Shroff on the other hand used one spare embryo from her own IVF programme to create her stem lines that she now injects into her patients. Her breakthrough has been reported in the media nationally and internationally including the UK's *Guardian* and Sky News network and she is possibly the only scientist in the world today who has made a successful transition from extraction to insertion with demonstrable biovalue (in the shape of use value) as her only validation and proof. Despite domestic and international media casting aspersions on her methods, technique and indeed casting her in a predefined and available category of the maverick anomalous scientist, she remains committed to her patients who have in turn developed an almost devotional attachment to her, their saviour. Even the most sceptical of media reports could not overlook the fact that fathers were breaking down at the sight of their paralysed child taking their first tentative steps in 11 sometimes 14 years; or an affluent London based NRI (non-resident Indian) suffering from rapidly advancing Motor Neuron Disease swallowing food and breathing without any assistance since her biocrossing to India a year ago. What is happening is clearly in the realm of fiction now seemingly realised and defies all 'rational' thought process the moderns are enjoined to embrace. However Dr Shroff is no saint, in fact she is a woman doing science dominated by men, an Indian in the world led by the United States and a human with real material ambitions. This is indeed ironic despite the rise of neoIndia on the global stage (Bharadwaj, 2006c). The reason her breakthrough is not adequately peer reviewed and validated by the international community is primarily because she finds the process of transcending from having successfully generated use value to creating exchange value very difficult. A private individual, warding off domestic and international pressure, with her pool of 200 bioavailable patients who in turn have all but surrendered their bodies to her scientific breakthrough, her only remaining concern is how to protect her intellectual property in a globalised research system. Rightly or wrongly she fears the scientific world will be quick to discredit her and walk away with her scientific gains. There are good reasons why she continues to be sceptical about sharing her breakthrough. The drama is unfolding on a daily basis. Sky News ran another report within weeks after breaking the story. As the scrutiny accentuates it is quite possible that Dr Shroff and her patients will be quarantined by the Indian state. The Indian government is busy rushing new legislation through parliament with the view, at least in principle, to control better the research and application of embryonic stem cells in the country. Once these laws come into effect it is likely Dr Shroff will either be forced to shut down or barred from recruiting any new patients.[6] Perhaps we can hope to see a biosocial rising as her patients and similar others demand access to a potentially 'dangerous' and experimental stem cell therapy, which, for the moment, seems to work. However, informal conversations with many patients and their families indicates that they do not so much predicate their discourse on their biological biographies but rather around a woman who is able to offer promise of health, hope and healing. Therefore should there be a biosocial mobilisation actors will rise and congregate around a 'maverick' woman scientist, a *devi* or goddess to many, who bestows the gift of life rather than a mere scientist in a white coat. There are early signs that she is already being seen as a *devi*, which opens a Pandora's box of cultural analysis and gendered explanations. However even in the event of such an uprising it is highly problematic to conceptualise charismatic authority and beseeching supplication from patients as an instance of biosociality. As I argue elsewhere, it is not uncommon for science and religion to forge a symbiotic relationship in Indian IVF laboratories and for physicians/clinicians to be viewed and revered as life giving, sustaining and destroying deities (Bharadwaj, 2006b). In the IVF clinical and laboratory spaces it is fairly routine for Indian scientists and clinicians to display overt religiosity and enlist divine assistance in the process of high tech conception (ibid.). Unlike the Euro-American 'postmoderns' the Indian scientists and patients turn to more techno-science to overcome their fate while continuing to rail against the unyielding 'gods' (cf. Rabinow, 1996: 103). The concept of biosociality therefore fails to capture the place of the *supernatural* both as cultural practice and as experience of the 'uncanny', 'pre-objective' unknown (cf. Throop, 2005). The very act of petitioning the state and the resultant politicisation of the individuals, on the other hand, bypasses the biosociality question as well. Demands for relief and access to resources by drawing attention to the pain as 'the price of belonging to a society' – especially where such demands challenge the certainty of bureaucratically defined medical science – have in the past only transformed victims/patients/sufferers in India into mere 'malingerers' (cf. Das, 1995: 137–74) as opposed to biosocial actors.

Conclusion

For very different and difficult reasons both IVF and stem cell clinical trial patients in India and elsewhere have endured biocrossings, extractions and insertions. In so doing they remain biosocially inactive, inert, indifferent. This is hardly surprising at one level because so long as we live in a world where the poor, the unfit, the gendered, the stigmatised – to name a few problematic categories – are not so much 'killed', but rather 'allowed to die' (Das and Poole, 2004), concepts like biosociality will have to work very hard to explain both the idea of bio and the nature of sociality. This is not to claim that biosociality does not exist in India but rather the social trajectory of the bio and its biographical inscription seldom produces individual or group identities.

I have tried to argue that relatively poor and sick as well as prosperous but sick bodies in Indian IVF and stem cell labs are seldom biosocial but rather always bioavailable for biocrossings. To overlook this is to overlook the social and health inequalities across cultures and the differing opportunities for action and expression such inequalities engender. The poor in a neo-liberal world inhabit biologies that are routinely construed, following Nancy Scheper-Hughes (2000), as waste and I would argue further gain meaning only when such waste can be recycled in any tangible, meaningful and above all profitable sense. Thompson argues that in the 'biomedical mode of reproduction' unlike the capitalist mode of production, waste is seldom a political or logistical problem but rather an ethical one of how to designate life material (embryos) as waste (Thompson, 2005: 264). I am suggesting that in the neoliberal mode of production this problem is frequently addressed by resorting to recycling socially/ethically defined waste or surplus that cannot otherwise be gainfully accumulated. Through modern transplant technology the 'biosociality' of a few, Scheper-Hughes argues, is made possible through the literal incorporation of the body parts of those who often have no social destiny other than premature death (Scheper-Hughes, 2000). The same argument can be made for gendered and other kinds of marked bodies that die real and social deaths since either their bodies are deemed unimportant, unsalvageable or simply substitutable. A biocrossing therefore is a crossing made in a social space fraught with opportunity and danger which on occasions can be a calculated risk or a forced dislocation as the last resort.

I began this discussion alluding to the question of agency and its relationship to structure. While individuals and collectivities (as numerous anthropological and sociological studies have shown) seldom passively submit to the brutalising effects of power/knowledge, my personal ethnographic disquiet has always centred on the question what, if at all, is politically achieved from resisting and often passively? For example the model of passive suffering Indian womanhood or the Hindu ideology of *pativrata* or literally, she who takes a vow (*vrat*) of devotion to her husband (*pati*) (Harlan and Courtright, 1995: 8) was clearly instilled in the ancient religious laws of *Manu*, which still hold considerable sway over Indian women (Dhruvaranjan, 1989). Whilst such an ideological conformity might be the only available resource for some women trying to survive, negotiate, bargain, compromise and secure concessions, dispensations, extensions or exemptions, it nevertheless leaves the patriarchal structure fundamentally challenged but unaltered. However, resistance – of the brutalised, the weak and the infirm – can alter the structure at some rudimentary level remaking the conceptual boundaries of institutions like the state through the very act of securing survival and seeking justice from the margins (Das and Poole, 2004). That said, such altered structures seldom lose their power to code certain kinds of knowledges about individuals, populations and incompliant bodies or even tolerate the dilution of their ability to police, patrol and punish transgressions of dominant cultural norms and ideas. For example let us consider the issue of identities as rooted in agency. It is an anthropological truism that identities are multiple, complex, contextual, contingent and sometimes consensual. As identity forming resource, biosociality enables people to congregate around some aspect of their (failing) biology. In the everyday local moral worlds of patients and their carers however it is not so much identity issues that frame actions but rather life shaped by demands for resources and treatment, a cry for help, or a relentless but exhausting search for resolution. In the Indian context this entails forging of tactical alliances within and outside families as well as alliances born out of everyday emotional work of care giving (Bharadwaj, 2003). According to Das (2001) alignments between family and state embody a 'politics of domesticity, which involve connected body selves' and not liberal biosocial individuals in India (cited in Roberts, this volume). Equally Das also disallows any scope for entertaining the idea that the family and the community are more protective of the self than other collectivities ... [since] finely woven structures of power within the family often determine the level at which ill health of different members will be tolerated (Das, 1990: 43–5).

In other words there are those who suffer in silence but show resolve or openly resist with great tenacity but never develop a sense of identity other than those socially received or ascribed (e.g. the inauspicious barren woman, the emasculated infertile man, the senile, the invalid, the leper etc.). These identity ascriptions in turn may be negotiated/resisted individually or through a network of familial kin but seldom challenged to a point of total rejection.

Battaglia (1995) citing Strathern (1988) contends agent or acting subject may thus be less a locus for relationships than a 'pivot of relationships ... one who from his or her own vantage point acts with another in mind'. Agency thus approached can perhaps distil how the agents get farmed in relationships, exchanges and interactions. The unquestioned submission of the daughter-in-law in the IVF clinic or that of hopeless search for conception by Sumita and Shankar or indeed countless bioavailable bodies in stem cell trials are all examples of active agents working within limitations set by relationships, resources, ideologies and normative expectations. These struggles point to the definite limits to an idea of agency as even in the mode of resistance the actions, strategies, subversions can amount to no more than weaponry wielded by the weak (Scott, 1985). However, power relations and knowledge practices like cultures that contain them don't hold still for their portraits (Clifford and Marcus, 1986). Resistance and critique however passive produce eventual change, facilitate recoding of knowledge practices and realign power relations. This is seldom without a cost and inevitable social suffering. In this context it is worth revisiting Shankar and Sumita's contention who see 'social change' as 'law of nature' suggesting that 'everything in nature (*Prakriti*) changes including the customs, traditions, attitudes but to stand up against the contemporary norms is impossible, you have to conform'. Shankar and Sumita unlike their Euro-American counterparts have access to a cosmology that does not 'other' nature as a domain from which human intervention is absent. In this cosmogony to be nature (*Prakriti*) is to remain in a symbiotic relationship with the human (*Purush*) and subject to human industry and action (*Purshartha*).[7] Hence as with all things living, growth, change and movement is inevitable. The only impediments and obstacles in this worldview however are the torturous growth pains that mortal resistance to change brings.

Acknowledgements

Many thanks to Sahra Gibbon and Carlos Novas for their thought provoking and generous comments on this chapter. I am truly indebted to a number of colleagues, friends and biosociality workshop participants for their comments, suggestions and encouragement. A very special thank you to Nina Hallowell, Sarah Franklin, Janet Carsten and Marcia Inhorn.

Notes

1 Most notably when the essentialist ethno models of physiology and understanding of 'biology' as rooted in the paradigm of the biosciences and that of human (Cartesian) physiology collide in a contested field of cross-cultural (re)presentation.
2 Charis Thompson (2001), however, offers a brilliant critical departure from this position. Also see Janet Carsten (2004).
3 I am very aware that the Euro-American category is no less problematic than the category of 'the Indian'. I use this term as it has become normalised in anthropological literature and to refer to the collectivities and formations in Europe and North America and not as an 'othering' trope. The question of biosociality within the Euro-American

formation is fraught with complexities and difference. However whilst the idea of biosocial mobilisation in Europe and America is both conceptually and empirically thinkable, in global locales like India the concept remains problematic.

4 The biological must be understood in the broadest sense. Especially in the way it has become routinised in English language and everyday usage as well as a signifier for the human body and its internal/external functions and attributes that may have specific and contingent cultural/historical meanings. One such meaning can be gleaned in the discipline of the biosciences and the disciplinary modalities of biomedicine just as in multiple cross-cultural descriptions of human body and its various attributes. As a concept I am attempting to understand the 'biological' as a semiotic entity rather than reduced to a narrow cultural conception of the kind that has become linked to the bio-genetic language associated with the notion of the human in the bioscience paradigm. This polysemy is a valuable part of the 'situated' biographical inscription I am suggesting.

5 The data in this segment are drawn from multi-sited ethnographic research examining the clinical and lived experience of infertility and assisted conception in five Indian cities. The research was carried out from 1996 to 2001 and follow-up field work from 2003 to 2004.

6 Dr Shroff, however, is fighting back and finally taking steps to publish her research findings and seeking to protect her intellectual property by patenting her stem cell extraction and insertion technique she pioneered in her small research lab in Delhi.

7 There are four Pursharthas: Dharma (Righteous/Virtuous Conduct), Artha (Generation of Wealth), Kama (Pleasure, Desire and Regeneration) and Moksha (Liberation from Worldly Cycles of Birth and Death). The *Purush* (Man)/*Prakriti* (Nature) symbiosis is encoded with a distinct patriarchal bias. At a meta-level this union underscores a 'primordial' epochal procreative theory of creation wherein the hetero-normative male and female principals come together to reproduce and bring forth change and difference. In practical terms this amounts to nature (*Prakriti*) being made/extended/ modified through human action (*Purush/Purshartha*) just as human action is shaped/ curtailed/facilitated by a dynamic Nature (*Prakriti*).

References

Battaglia, Debbora (ed.) (1995) *Rhetorics of Self-Making*. Berkeley, CA: University of California Press.

Bharadwaj, Aditya (2001) *Conceptions: An Exploration of Infertility and Assisted Conceptions in India,* PhD thesis, University of Bristol.

Bharadwaj, Aditya (2003) Why Adoption is not an Option in India: The Visibility of Infertility, the Secrecy of Donor Insemination, and other Cultural Complexities', *Social Science and Medicine*, 56: 1867–80.

Bharadwaj, Aditya (2005) Cultures of Embryonic stem cell Research in India. In Bender, W., Hauskeller, C. and Manzei, A. (eds) *Crossing Borders: Cultural, Religious and Political Differences Concerning Stem Cell Research*. Münster: Agenda Verlag.

Bharadwaj, Aditya (2006a) Clinical Theodicies: The Enchanted World of Uncertain Science and Clinical Conception in India. *Culture Medicine and Psychiatry*, 30(4) (December).

Bharadwaj, Aditya (2006b) Contentious Liminalities: Embryonic Stem Cell Research in India and the UK. BIOS Seminar Series, London School of Economics and Political Studies, London, February.

Bharadwaj, Aditya (2006c) Reproductive Viability and the State: The Rise of Embryonic Stem Cells in India. Paper presented at Reproduction, Globalization and the State Conference. Rockefeller Foundation Bellagio Study and Conference Centre, Italy.

Bharadwaj, Aditya, Atkinson, Paul and Clarke, Angus (2006) Classification and the Experience of Genetic Haemochromatosis. In Atkinson, Paul and Glasner, Peter (ed.) *New Genetics, New Identities*. London: Routledge.

Carsten, Janet (2004) *After Kinship*. Cambridge: Cambridge University Press.

Clifford, James and Marcus, George. E. (eds) (1986) *Writing Cultures: The Poetics and Politics of Ethnography*. Berkeley, CA: University of California Press.

Cohen, Lawrence (2004) Operability: Surgery at the Margin of the State. In Das, Veena and Poole Deborah (ed.) *Anthropology in the Margins of the State*. Santa Fe, NM: SAR Press.

Cohen, Lawrence (2005) Operability, Bioavailability, and Exception. In Ong, Aihwa and Collier, Stephen, J. (ed.) *Global Assemblages: Technology, Politics, and Ethics as Anthropological Problems*. Oxford: Blackwell Publishing.

Das, Veena (1990) What do we mean by Health? In Caldwell, John and Fendley, Sally (eds) *In Health Transition Volume II*. Canberra: Australian National University.

Das, Veena (1995) Suffering, Legitimacy and Healing: The Bhopal Case. In *Critical Events: An Anthropological Perspective on Contemporary India*. Delhi: Oxford University Press.

Das, Veena and Poole, Deborah (2004) State and Its Margins: Comparative Ethnographies. In Das, Veena and Poole Deborah (eds) *Anthropology in the Margins of the State*. Santa Fe, NM: SAR Press.

Dhruvaranjan, Vanaja (1989) *Hindu Women and the Power of Ideology*. Gramby, MA: Bergin and Garvey.

Farmer, Paul (2003) *Pathologies of Power: Health, Human Rights, and the New War on the Poor*. Berkeley, CA: University of California Press.

Franklin, Sarah (2003) Ethical Biocapital: New Strategies of Cell Culture. In Franklin, S. and Lock, M. (eds) *Remaking Life and Death: Towards an Anthropology of the Biosciences*. Santa Fe, NM: School of American Research Press.

Haraway, Donna (1990) A Manifesto for Cyborgs: Science, Technology, and Socialist Feminism in the 1980s. In Nicholson, L. J (ed.) *Feminism/Postmodernism*. London: Routledge.

Haraway, D. (1991) *Simians, Cyborgs and Women: The Reinvention of Nature*. New York: Routledge.

Harlan, Lindsey and Courtright, Paul B. (eds) (1995) *From the Margins of Hindu Marriage: Essays on Gender, Religion and Culture*. New York: Oxford University Press.

Inhorn, Marcia (2003) *Making Muslim Babies: Gender, Science, and In Vitro Technologies in Egypt*. New York: Routledge.

Inhorn, Marcia and Bharadwaj, Aditya (2006) Reproductively Disabled Lives: Infertility, Stigma and Suffering in Egypt and India. In Ingstad, B. and Whyte, S. R. (with Inhorn, M.) (eds) *Disability in Local and Global Worlds*. Berkeley, CA: University of California Press (in press).

Latour, B. (1993) *We Have Never Been Modern*. Cambridge, MA: Harvard University Press.

Marx, K. (1963) *Capital*, Volume 1, Moscow: Progress Publisehrs.

Nichter, Mark and Nichter, Mimi (1996) *Anthropology and International Health: Asian Case Studies*, 2nd edn. Amsterdam: Gordon and Breach.

Ong, A. and Collier, S. (ed.) (2005) *Global Assemblages. Technology, Politics and Ethics as Anthropological Problems*, Oxford: Blackwell.

Rabinow, Paul (1992) Artificiality and Enlightenment: From Sociobiology to Biosociality. In Crary, J. and Kwinter, S. (eds) *Incorporations*. New York: Zone.

Rabinow, Paul (1996) Artificiality and Enlightenment: From Sociobiology to Biosociality. In *Essays on the Anthropology of Reason*. Princeton, NJ: Princeton University Press.

Rapp, Rayna (2000) Extra Chromosomes and Blue Tulips: Medico-Familial Interpretations. In Lock, Margaret, Young, Allan and Cambrosio, Alberto (eds) *Living and Working with the New Medical Technologies: Intersections of Inquiry.* Cambridge: Cambridge University Press.

Rose, Nikolas and Novas, Carlos (2005) Biological Citizenship. In Aihwa Ong and Stephen J. Collier (eds) *Global Assemblages: Technology, Politics, and Ethics as Anthropological Problems*. Oxford: Blackwell.

Scheper-Hughes, Nancy (2000) The Global Traffic in Human Organs. *Current Anthropology*, 41(2): 191–224.

Scott, James, C. (1985) *Weapons of the Weak: Everyday Forms of Peasant Resistance*. New Haven, CT: Yale University Press.

Strathern, Marilyn (1988) *The Gender of the Gift: Problems with Women and Problems with Society in Melanesia*. Berkeley, CA: University of California Press.

Strathern, Marilyn (1992) *Reproducing the Future: Anthropology, Kinship and the New Reproductive Technologies*. New York: Routledge.

Thompson, Charis (2001) Strategic Naturalizing: Kinship in an Infertility Clinic. In Franklin, Sarah and Mckinnon, Susan (ed.) *Relative Values: Reconfiguring Kinship Studies*. Durham, NC and London: Duke University Press.

Thompson, Charis (2005) *Making Parents: The Ontological Choreography of Reproductive Technologies*. Cambridge, MA: MIT Press.

Throop, Jason C. (2005) Hypocognition, a 'Sense of the Uncanny', and the Anthropology of Ambiguity: Reflections on Robert I. Levy's Contribution to Theories of Experience in Anthropology. *Ethos*, 33(4): 499–511.

UNICEF (2006) http://www.unicef.org/.

Waldby, Catherine (2002) Stem Cells, Tissue Cultures and the Production of Biovalue. *Health*, 6(3): 305–23.

6 Synecdochic ricochets

Biosocialities in a Jerusalem IVF clinic

Michal Nahman

This essay is an attempt to think through and employ the concept of biosociality ethnographically. I begin this with a discussion of the concept of biosociality itself, then explore how this can be worked through Donna Haraway's notion of "cyborg politics" (1991) and how that helps me to engage with the research material I've brought to this conversation. It moves ethnographically to a statement made by a key research participant in my study of Israeli ova donation. This is then used to frame three ethnographic biosocial moments in the practices of human ova extraction, exchange and implantation in an Israeli IVF clinic in Jerusalem. What emerges is a discussion of the politics of life and death in Israel (Foucault 1978). In so doing I explore how biosociality helps me to sustain a politically engaged and situated analysis of Israeli reproduction in a time of war.

Biosociality as I understand it has three dimensions. The first sense in which it was invoked by Rabinow, it seems, is to suggest the way that epistemologies of culture and nature are imploding. This first sense of the term indicates that older ways on understanding culture, which relied on a modeling of culture on nature, are obsolete. Nowadays, with emergent technological practices, "nature [is] known and remade through technique and will finally become artificial" (Rabinow 1995: 99). In this sense, it is no longer sufficient to rely on a view of "nature" and the "natural" that is uninterrogated (Haraway 1997; Franklin *et al.* 2000). Instead, nature itself is being recast in terms of cultural references. Artificiality, then, encompasses both nature and culture.

The notion of making nature artificial can be thought of in terms of IVF as a technology for making "artificial" kin relations. In a broader sense, one can think of larger collectivities as being founded "artificially" (as has been well established through the notion of "imagined communities [Anderson 1983]). In the case of the state of Israel, this is particularly relevant. The very recent inception of the state requires much rhetorical and ideological work to naturalize the connection between the body, the individual, the nation, religion and the homeland. Mobilizations of arguments about historical links of Jews to the biblical land of Israel, and contemporary naturalization of processes of Israel state expansion are two examples in this multifarious process. This discussion will be returned to below, when I present an ethnographic example of "embryo transfer," which can be metaphorically thought of in relation to the politics of media discussions about transferring Palestinians out of the West Bank – ethnic cleansing – and also materially, in terms of Israeli state demographic policies and practices – in terms of work done to discourage Palestinian reproduction, and to promote Jewish reproduction.

The second sense in which Rabinow invokes his notion of biosociality indicates the new kinds of relations between individual and state that emerge in the practices of science and technology. Here, as I understand it, he is referring to new kinds of collectivities or "assemblages" which form in relation to diseases. In some cases, as is demonstrated by some of the authors in this volume, patient advocacy and activism are being formed to cope with new ontologies in the world. Now that science "enables" us to see further and further into bodies, individuals and groups have a stake in harnessing this ability, advocating their role as decision makers and enacting new kinds of citizenship. This second sense emerges in my research in a more diffuse way, in that the ethnographic examples below indicate new and old articulations between the citizen and the state (both the biopower of managing populations and bodies; and the old sovereign power to "dispose" of life). Here I bring in the ideas of Foucault (1978) and Agamben (1995) regarding life, its disposability and how this enacts particular kinds of old and new state power.

The third sense in which I understand this concept of biosociality is in terms of ethnographic ways of knowing about the world. In *French DNA* (1999) Rabinow articulates this well, arguing that the role of the ethnographer is "nominalist" (p. 180). He states, "[a] sensibility of constant change, and a certain pleasure and obligation to grasp it and participate in the transformations, constitute one mode of relating to things" (1999: 181). To name, identify and witness emergences in the biosciences as one central aspect of the ethnography of knowledge, I attempt to foreground this issue. By employing a feminist textual strategy of "synecdochic ricochet" (which is explained below) I hope to enact this third dimension of ethnographic biosociality, which I see as being about drawing together often disparate events, individuals, sets of politics and practices into a biosocial ethnographic assemblage. This assemblage plays on Rabinow's notion of the artificiality of nature and culture that now determines the post-enlightenment era in which we write and produce knowledge about people and practices.

Synecdoche: while working my way through these ideas ethnographically I employ a mixture of approaches to grasp, name and evaluate the situations in which ova extraction, exchange and implantation occur. As such, this chapter does not critique biosociality as much as employ it as an approach to understanding ontological and epistemological questions in ethnographic research of IVF in Israel. A range of further approaches is drawn from the anthropology, political theory and feminist technoscience studies. What I map out are different synecdochal moments that connect up Israeli state-making practices with biomedical baby-making practices: kinds of biosocial moments.

Ricochet: practices of extracting, fertilizing and implanting ova are seen in this paper as a site of ricochet between technique and the state (Hayden 1995). Biosociality is at play in diffuse ways that are illustrated by ethnographic examples that highlight the rupture, reaffirmation, and rearticulation of "the national" (borders, bodies and ideals). This also indicates shifting relations between the individual and the state. Attention to these sites of articulation of biomedical practices, state policy and social relations, facilitates a meditation on the kinds of relations and relationalities now emerging between the state and body parts of its citizens. Inspiration is drawn from Rabinow's (1999) illustration of how practices and politicization of the Human Genome Project have remade the relations between the individual, DNA, organizations and the state. This rearticulation also happens in ways that are not always direct.

While these relations are being reassembled, what is the nature of the relations themselves? How do the practices, people, emotions and body parts get connected up with one another?

Cyborg politics

The concept of biosociality is powerful in its wide ranging possibility for thinking not only about culture but also about the practices of producing culture through ethnographic writing. Likewise, Haraway (1991) argued against totalizing theories of society, while attending to the issues of capital and labour from Marxist and socialist feminist perspectives. For her this involves making fictions that draw *potent connections*, which reveal the "truth" about practices and knowledges. Haraway enjoins,

> One important route … is through theory and practice addressed to the social relations of science and technology, including crucially the systems of myth and meanings structuring our imaginations. The cyborg is a kind of disassembled and reassembled, postmodern collective and personal self. This is the self feminists must code.
>
> (Haraway 1991: 163)

Far from being solely about the way in which technology and humans are now somehow merged, cyborg writing is about creative feminist renderings of (what feminism is and) the world of technology, the body, global capitalism and history which maps, our social and bodily reality as an imaginative resource suggesting some very fruitful couplings (Haraway 1991: 150).

The strategy of cyborg writing, of assemblage and reassemblage, and of fruitful couplings is employed in this chapter in order to construct a story about borders, bodies and body parts in Israel, that provides a witnessing of the way history, state agendas and micropractices of the body cohere. My mode of doing this is through "synecdochic ricochet." The various "ricochets" exemplified in the stories below are intended to evoke coherent versions of the present day political practices of reproduction in Israel. The typical language of benevolence, pro-natality, and survival that is often associated with Israeli reproduction is critiqued as part of a wider feminist critique of such approaches (Yuval-Davis 1997; Kanaaneh 2002).

The stories below are presented as fieldnotes. They were compiled and drawn from notes I wrote in three different notebooks, and in emails to my friends and my doctoral advisor while I was conducting research in Israel in 2002. My use of the figurational strategy of a synecdoche between extraction, exchange and implantation of eggs and settlement, transfer, and guarding of nations is a way of drawing attention to connections between bodies and government, self and collectivity, and self and other. I use this mode of analysis as a way of critiquing political state Zionism and particular forms of biopower. In this sense, "synecdoche" figures a relationship between the stuff of bodies and the powers of governing subjects. Without essentializing the kinds of bodies in question (e.g. I do not assert that "women" reproduce "families" or "nations"), I suggest that synecdochal relations occur in various ways in the discursive practices of ovum extraction, exchange, fertilization and implantation; this is done in order to assert that subjects are materialized through the relations which are produced by exchanges, extractions, manipulations, and legal debates about bodies and body parts. The discursive practices of ova extraction, fertilization, implantation and exchange are condensed nodes which produce and are produced by the nation – in a feminist poststructuralist sense, they materialize one another.

The research drawn on for this paper comes from a study I conducted during the early days of the building of a wall between Israel and the West Bank, as well as during the second Palestinian intifada, between January and September 2002, so the practices of ova extraction and exchange are inevitably contextualized in this, having occurred almost literally at the foot of the wall. The "synecdochic ricochets" therefore characterize not only the kinds of biosociality that are taking place in the discursive practices of Israeli ova extraction, exchange and implantation, but also the kind of politics that can be done through cyborg writing and the highlighting of biosocial ethnographic moments. It is the connection between war, bullets, apartheid walls, martyrdom, gender, race, class, ova extraction and embryo transfer that is being evoked.

Context: ova donation, intifada and the Israeli health care system

Ova donation has been practiced in Israel since 1984.[1] In 1987 legislation on IVF came into effect dictating the legality of egg donation, in cases where the donor woman was an IVF patient. This practice remains in effect. In parallel with this, Israeli IVF physicians have been building on existing links with doctors in Romania, Cyprus, Spain, the Czech Republic and the USA, promoting transnational egg donation. In transnational egg donation, physicians "prepare" their Israeli patients hormonally for "embryo transfer" and then Israeli women travel abroad to be implanted with ova (Nahman 2006).[2]

The practices of transnational donation are enabled by Israel's two-tiered medical system. All Israeli physicians are employed by one of the national "sick funds" or *kupot holim*. They spend a certain amount of time practicing medicine in state-run hospitals. In addition to this, physicians may practice at private institutions where individuals pay for treatments not covered under their "health basket" (the types of treatments covered by the sick funds are listed under each sick fund's *sal briut* – health basket). It is through the private institutions that Israeli ova donation moves out of Israel's borders to other countries.

In 1994, the Israeli Parliament enacted the National Health Insurance bill (NHI). However, Israeli health reforms existed for most of the state's history, long before reform in other Western states (Chernichovsky and Chinitz 1995). This reform was enacted to expand access and medical rights. It shifted the management of healthcare from the domain of the state to the domain of sick funds administered through government hospitals. These changes were made at the same time as reforms in other countries such as the UK, the Netherlands and New Zealand and were different,

> according to their cultural, social, historical and political circumstances. Even so, the economic and organizational issues are the same everywhere: how to contain costs, increase efficiency, satisfy consumers and providers, achieve equity, and improve the quality of health care.
>
> (Chernichovsky 1992)

The specificity of the Israeli situation is worth noting. This 1994 shift, occurred just in the aftermath of the first 1987–92 Palestinian intifada, which had a significant impact on the state's economic stability (Fielding 2003: 5 n5). These shifts in the health system, divesting the government of direct management of the health system were deeply embedded in the political changes and associated economic instability.

Alongside the NHI was the emergence of private health insurance, which people could opt into. Private medical services were being offered in private hospitals and soon patients could pay out of pocket for treatments (usually with elite physicians) in public medical institutions (Shirom 2001: 325). Thus the "nationalizing" of the health system in effect split and mixed it into many different branches being administered by different bodies, some of which are nationally funded by the national sick funds and others which are not. Given that Israel has not traditionally had a privatized medical system, this privatization is having effects that are being felt in many areas of medicine. This was made clear to me through my interviews with patients, physicians and health advocates (see Nahman n.d.). Thus, some new sociocultural relations and practices are emerging in Israel in terms of these changes to access.

These shifts have ricocheted into practices of egg donation. They take many different forms, as indicated above, including transnational egg donation. These cultural ricochets of the changes in the healthcare system are particularly salient in the case of ova donation since this reproductive practice opens up fundamental questions not only of motherhood and relationality, but also of (biological) citizenship and nationality (Novas and Rose 2005).

Demographic issues: reproducing the Israeli state as Jewish

In contemporary Israel, the question of who is the mother in egg donation, as I found in my study, is fundamentally connected to questions about the reproduction of the state as Jewish. It has been noted already that exploring Israeli IVF involves thinking about how Jews think about relatedness, whether that is connected to gestation or to genetics (Kahn 2000). Coupled with this, it is important to note how Palestinians and other non-Jews, as well as marginalized Jews think of relatedness. In egg donation, some bodies become classed as Jewish or non-Jewish; Israeli or non-Israeli.

Crucially, Israeli citizenship (that is citizenship in which rights and access to state resources are realizable in daily life)[3] partly depends on a person being designated as Ashkenazi/European Jewish. One way in which the state realizes this biopolitical goal of making more Jewish citizens is through demographic management of the population (Foucault 1978). The survival of the state has traditionally been framed by its leaders as being dependent on the survival of the Jewish nation[4] and on reproduction. The importance of demography was underscored by the Israeli government already in 1968 with the establishment of the Demographic Center (Portugese 1998: 77). The aim of this centre was to,

> act systematically in carrying out a natality policy … such that natality will be encouraged and stimulated, an increase in natality in Israel being crucial for the whole future of the Jewish people.
>
> (cited in Portugese 1998: 77)

There were other natal policies relevant to Palestinians. However, generally these were aimed at the discouragement of reproduction (see Kanaaneh 2002). Jewish pronatalism was therefore inscribed in the policies and practices of state institutions such as the Demographic Center.

There has been a recent resurgence in concern about demography in Israel, with several research centres producing statistics on ways to maintain the Jewish character of the state. Within practices and policies of reproduction this can be seen in the Israeli state subsidies of egg donation (within Israel) for women aged 45–51. This subsidy is unlimited until the conception and birth of one child (Rabinerson *et al.* 2002). A study conducted of this age group, across two years, with a sample of 254 Israeli women, found that the "success rate" (meaning the number of babies born) was 17.7% (ibid.). Despite these low success rates, Israel continues to subsidize ova donation. Given the state's history of aggressive pronatalism (Yuval-Davis 1989, 1997; Portugese 1998; Kanaaneh 2002) it seems that ova donation, too, is part of this state project.

Yet geographic expansion has increasingly been a concern and an integral aspect to the securing of the borders of the state. One major aspect of this has been the euphemistic suggestion that Palestinians be transferred out of Israeli occupied territories. This suggestion for ethnic cleansing was replayed by state representatives on the Israeli news in 2002 when my research was conducted.

Further suggestions were that a separation plan be put in place (Galili 2005). The idea of separation involved building a wall along the Green line separating Israel from the West Bank. The repetition of these ideas on Israeli news helped naturalize the idea of a coherent and separate Israeli state and a coherent and separate Palestinian home in the West Bank and Gaza.

Yet, while this separation has already come into effect with the removal of Jewish settlements from Gaza and the creation of a wall along the West Bank, two kinds of borders have been carved out. The first is a symbolic border along a newly imagined green line (one which is different from the 1967 border, and which splits apart Palestinian villages), materially realized by what the Israeli Left is calling the apartheid wall. The second is a dispersed border, which spreads web-like across the West Bank, dotted with checkpoints.

While the concrete borders of the state are mapped out in these ways, borders of reproduction are also web-like, made through practices and policies aimed at Palestinians, and Mizrakhi and Ashkenazi Jews. A striking example of such differential relations of women to reproduction practices of the state is that of the image of pregnant Palestinians awaiting passage at a checkpoint on route to a hospital and being forced to give birth at the checkpoint, whilst hiding from Israeli soldiers (Levy 2003). Also, whilst the Israeli healthcare system was meant to ensure access for all to health services free of charge,

> In the State of Israel in 2006, women live, fall ill and die because of a lack of medical insurance and the economic means necessary to be cured.
>
> (Levy 2006)

In his article in the left-leaning Israeli newspaper Ha'aretz, journalist Gideon Levy presents the case of marginal women born in Israel who do not experience Israel's liberal national health services in the way they should, precisely because they do not fall into the category of proper citizens.

In the case of Israeli IVF and ova donation, the borders of citizenship are made along more religious lines. Despite the fact that rabbinical leaders decided that ova do not challenge the status of the birth mother, a new law which was written and proposed to the Israeli parliament in 2001, will make it illegal to donate ova between people of different religious faiths. Hence, the rabbinical reasoning, which can be summed up as, gestation-not-genetics-makes-the-kinship-bond, is coming into question in light of contemporary political pressures to maintain the Jewish character of the state. These are important nodes that are integral to the story of the biopolitics of reproduction in Israel.

A perceptible tension exists between explanations of geographic expansionism and demographic increase of the population. Inherent to both are contradictions about state support versus outcomes, and the complexity of the kinds of borders and boundaries created. I return to this below.

How "the national" was brought into the clinic

"Making more disposable people"

Daily observations of doctor–patient consultations formed a large part of this part of the study. Such meetings were characterized by the patient entering the office, sitting down and having a discussion with the physician, then leaving with instructions to speak to the nurse or the secretary. After each successive patient/couple left, Professor Biton, the head of the IVF unit at this Jerusalem clinic would provide commentary to me on what had transpired. His details involved information about IVF practices, and also seemingly unrelated details about patients' lives. His remarks were often paternalistic and illustrative of his investment in the success of his "cases."

On one particularly notable occasion, as we discussed why the health system pays for so many IVF cycles, Biton explained to me (tongue in cheek) that this is in order, "to make more disposable people." He then retracted this statement. It may be that Biton's "joke" about "making more disposable people" was part of the "unfunny wit" through which people express anxieties about their society's boundaries (Douglas 1966: 147). Mary Douglas delineates four kinds of "social pollution" through which a society expresses concerns over its boundaries through humour. Biton's joke seems to express an anxiety about the fourth kind of "social pollution": "[D]anger from internal contradiction, when the basic postulates are denied by other basic postulates, so that at certain points the system seems to be at war with itself" (Douglas 1966: 146–7). In some cases, then, humor may be used to express anxiety over contradictions.

It has been argued that the Israeli state places great emphasis on producing more Jewish people, through pronatalist legislation, media representations and various other practices (Kahn 2000; Kanaaneh 2002; Portugese 1998; Yuval-Davis 1989, 1997). Yet, its expansionist and colonialist politics and military practices (Shafir 1999) mean that the Israeli state uses its citizens in a manner that "disposes" of them (through military incursions into Palestinian cities, and in this sense, "provoking" further violence).

The term "demographic race" or "demographic war" refers to one of the battlefields of the Israeli "war over home." One of the major threats to the existence of the state, *as an exclusively Jewish one*, is thought to be the "over-reproduction" of Palestinians. During research conducted in Israel in 2002, the "disposability" of Palestinians was hinted at by Israelis both in everyday life and on televised news programs. This notion of the over-reproduction of Palestinians (and concomitant Orientalist and racialized views of them as more primitive [Kanaaneh 2002]) has led to state policies which favor Jewish reproduction so that Jews will win the "demographic race" within the Israeli state. The state's "demographic race" against the Palestinians, along with its constant search for new and legitimate sources of immigration represent two aspects of the attention that is paid to maintaining the Jewish character of the state. [5] At the same time, the state expands its territory as it has done in the West Bank throughout the last few years. These two aspects may seem contradictory in the sense that the government enacts military practices and policies which endanger the very "Jewish nation" which it is said to be protecting.

Biton's joke about IVF practices being facilitated by the government in order to make more disposable people may express his anxiety about the contradictions between the state's financial and structural support (in the form of hospitals and programs) for IVF and its high investment in military activity. Mary Douglas suggests that humor displays an anxiety about the nation's borders and contradictions between what the state says and what it does. So "making more disposable people" could be signaling Biton's anxiety about the seeming contradictory nature of fostering life whilst allowing people to die in military actions and suicide bombings.

However, "making more disposable people" could be viewed in another way. Rather than expressing a solely psychological response of one person, this joke can be seen as a "material-semiotic generative node" (Haraway 1997) or a way of doing theory through the lay formulations of people (Strathern 1991; Verran 1998). This is fundamentally about the question of *which* life has greater value to the state. Notions of waste figure centrally to the classical anthropological canon, of so-called "primitive" societies. The Israeli framing of Palestinians as more primitive and therefore expendable fits in with this literature in the sense that certain kinds of pollution, sacrifice and waste are viewed in classical anthropology as ways of performing social relations and consolidating them (Mauss 1991 [1950]; Douglas 1966; Titmuss 1970; Hubert and Mauss 1964 [1899]). Arguably, then, the Israeli state is attempting to consolidate its status as a Euro-American power and this is being done not only through the management of the population, but also through the disposal of "bare life."

In other words, this notion of making more disposable people can be seen as a discursive moment that indexes biopolitics and the sovereign power to dispose of life. In Western history the sovereign has had the power to take a life (execution without sacrifice, as is outlined by Agamben in *Homo Sacer* 1995). Foucault (1978) argues that in the new era of biopolitics there is greater emphasis on the management of life (the population and of bodily discipline). Agamben (1995) extends and critiques Foucault by insisting on the centrality of the disposability of life and the creation of death in contemporary biopolitics. He does so through a notion of a juridical "state of exception" (borrowed from the work of Carl Schmitt), in which life is made legally expendable by making it extra-legal (see Butler 2004). Agamben argues that "psychological" interpretations (such as Douglas's perhaps) are insufficient (1995: 6).

Something more is going on here with Biton's assertion that IVF is about "making more disposable people." IVF is always about producing an excess of embryos. The processes of ovarian hyper-stimulation, ova fertilization, freezing of embryos and their implantation involves disposal at every stage. So in this case it is about disposal of "potential" people, what Thompson has called "promissory capital" (Thompson 2005). If a woman's ovary produces 20 ova, not all of these will be seen by the embryologist as "suitable" for fertilization; they might be seen as "too small," or their membrane "too permeable" or "soft." For example, if during the insertion of a sperm into an ovum the cell membrane is too pliable it is likely that an embryo will develop out of the fertilized ovum. Hence disposability is an integral part of IVF in general.

What makes this disposability pertinent to biopolitics and biosociality in the context of Israeli IVF is that this disposability is directly linked to the politics of maintaining the state and imaginaries of the nation. Seeing these connections means attending to the ways in which, "the realm of bare life gradually begins to coincide with the political realm" (Agamben 1995: 9). So rather than solely focusing on the way in which the state manages bodies and populations (biopower and biopolitics in the Foucauldian sense) Agamben is asking for an attention to the ways in which politics and the body slowly (and in specific moments in time) merge.

It is in this way that "making more disposable people" is also a kind of diffuse biosocial ethnographic moment. While Agamben is talking about a generalized political realm, Rabinow's "biosociality" is asking for attention to precisely those "moments" or "events" (1999: 181). Rabinow's crucial formulation is as follows,

> From time to time, and always in time, new forms emerge that catalyze previously existing actors, things, temporalities, or spatialities into a new mode of existence …
>
> (Rabinow 1999: 180)

The temporality which Rabinow is indicating here is crucial. Israeli IVF and national imaginaries are situated in a very particular historical and spatial moment and configuration.

Rabinow continues:

> Events problematize classifications, practices, things. The problematization of classifications, practices, things is an event.
>
> (Rabinow 1999: 181)

So, the disposability in "making more disposable people" is a temporally and geopolitically located discursive construction which enacts the relations between the state and the individual in several ways: recreating the old power of the state to dispose of people; connecting the techniques of IVF to the techniques of war; creating a space in which to think about and express the nation's borders. This is particularly relevant to the case of ova donation, which is an act of taking inside one's body something which was not there previously. In a sense, the Israeli government's populating of the West Bank (and its ability to extract its citizens from Gaza and some parts of the West Bank) with settlements can be taken as one more instance of this synecdochic connection.

Such a "moment" is a node in the webs of Israeli reproduction, through which making a Jewish person through egg donation and IVF becomes naturalized as part of a national war against an "Other." There is a scale switching occurring here in Biton's words where which, 'a small thing can be made to say as much as a "'big' thing" (Strathern 1991: xix). I see the phrase, "making more disposable people" as explicating connections between technique, ideas about the natural and the inherent character of the nation. It is what Strathern has called a node of a social relationship (Strathern 1991: 101).

According to Strathern, what should hold the attention of anthropologists are "the analogies people draw between the various relationships which constitute sociality for them" (1991: 103). The scaling performed by Biton in his comment is, as I have said, one of synecdoche. The part (the embryo or ovum) stands in for the whole (a disposable people). He and others I encountered in my research were so extremely disaffected by their government's claims to be protecting and securing them, while aggressively promoting a militaristic and expansionist agenda. One ovum recipient husband argued that he would not send his child to the army because the state had not subsidized his egg donation. Many individuals encountered in this research echoed Biton's words in different ways. They did so in ways which the individual body or microscopic body parts were meant to stand in for the nation – a Jewish body stood in for the Jewish nation, a Palestinian body stood in for the Palestinian nation, in the war of words and blame that took place in the year during which this research was conducted. Thus Biton's phrase is a kind of local expression of the kind of relationship being enacted between technique, bodily stuff and the nation. I am using this node to hold together other kinds of moments where technique naturalizes cultural practices of ova extraction, exchange, fertilization and implantation. In the following sections, ethnographic moments are examined and juxtaposed in a way that is meant to enact some of the complex links between militarism, gender, borders and reproduction that are hinted at in Biton's words.

Dikkur: the discursive violence of ova extraction

The first of these three biosocial encounters indicates how language carries violence into the bodies of women, through techniques of biomedicine.

Fieldnote

Extraction of ova is known here as a *dikkur* in Hebrew or "aspiration" in English. The first term, *dikkur*, is the one most commonly used in the clinic. The word literally means "a stabbing" or "a pricking." When Biton explains the procedure he says (in English this time) that he is literally stabbing the ovary. He jokingly tells me that he skewers the ovaries, as if they were a *shish kebab*.

As I watched countless *dikkur* procedures, Biton actually seemed extremely careful, and the procedure looks nothing like a stabbing. Yet this name suggests that getting eggs out of women's bodies is a violent practice, or that at least, violence is inherent to some aspects of this practice – if only in its culturally specific name. Tsippi Ivri (1999) has shown the extent to which the discursive practices of becoming a mother and giving birth in Israel are militarized. I read the naming practices in Israeli ova donation as militarized as well.

Yet there is another element relating to our discussion in this volume, which is that it naturalizes violence as part of assisted parenthood. The supposedly violent practice of extracting eggs could be contrasted with the more gentle popular culture representations of the practices of making babies which are often concerned with the reproduction of the family, couple, nation or "global village." And of course there is the name for it in English, aspiration, which relates to breath, life and hope (see Franklin 1997 on IVF as a "hope technology"). Yet, here, the discursive strategy of stabbing reverberates with the reference to war in Biton's statement that he was making disposable people. The connections and naturalizations between the individual and the collective, the natural and cultural can perhaps be better explicated in the following set of fieldnotes pertaining to embryo transfer, or the implantation of fertilized ova into women's bodies.

Treating the enemy

Fieldnote

I spent the day in the clinic, in and out of nurses' and physicians' offices, observing and talking to people. There were two television screens mounted on the walls of the waiting room, which were always tuned to the news. There in the clinic, when I was trying to concentrate on "new ways of creating life," one could not avoid the media images of bloody attacks and destroyed buses. Ilanit (one of the nurses) and I talked for a while about the depressing state of affairs. I asked her whether it changes how she relates to "Arab" patients. She says "no way," insisting that she treats them as individuals giving them the proper level of care. When I observe her with them she is clearly more guarded but very attentive, warm and helpful.

After chatting with Ilanit I observed a *dikkur* from inside the laboratory. I could hear the patient being anesthetized, the physician cleaning her and preparing for the procedure. During all of this, while the patient was falling asleep I overheard the staff in the surgery room talk about where the patient is from, "Hebron or Bethlehem?" It turned out to be the latter. The nurse said, "I checked it out, wanted to see if we're neighbors you know. I live in Efrat."[6] As the procedure continued and vials were passed into the laboratory where I sat, they joked about whether there would be a ceasefire to accommodate the Jewish holiday of Purim and the Muslim *"Kurban"* (sacrificial celebration) which coincided that year. Osnat was at the microscope, determining the number of eggs retrieved. Judy the *mashgikha*[7] was sitting by Nurit and Sarit, the other two embryologists. Osnat was having difficulty finding eggs. So Sarit joined her at the next microscope.

While examining the ova through the microscope Sarit chatted with me about how amazing it is to see the results of her IVF work when she picks up her daughter from kindergarten. At her daughter's school there are the children of couples whom she has done the laboratory work for in the IVF unit. She explains that she looks at these children and thinks, "I know you since you were under the microscope."

Quickly pouring liquid from the test tubes into Petri dishes the embryologists checked them under the microscope and found two oocytes. When these were found the embryologists labeled the dish (marking the relative location of the specimen) and stacked the Petri dishes. All the while they were still chatting.

Osnat makes a pun with the woman's name: "what's her name? Shaheen?" There was a pause. "Shahid"[8] she mumbled. The other embryologist chuckled. They separated the eggs, washing them of any blood or other fluids. They then manage the *rishoom*, the registration of all the information on a treatment record sheet which would be copied and placed in the patient file and the laboratory records. Sarit then told me that these eggs are very small, implying they may not be "viable." "Eggs must be kept in the incubator for a minimum amount of time," she added informatively. She then double checks each of the empty Petri dishes and disposes of them. The eggs are moved into the incubator where the space is labeled with the woman's name. She documents the time, number of eggs and the treating physician. The laboratory has a file for each patient. If there is an egg donation, this is marked on the sheet. Each egg to be donated is specially marked on the record sheet.

This patient's treatment appeared to be normal, and standard procedures were apparently followed. Yet, the talk while the woman was being put to sleep and while sorting her ova was about an imagined enemy. The talk seemed casual, quotidian; there was not an air of the unusual. The contrast between Sarit's talk about her daughter's friends at kindergarten (whom she fondly remembers from "under the microscope") and her talk about the smallness of Shaheen's "unviable" ova is striking. Osnat's pun on Shaheen's name may be one way in which techniques of extraction (of viable and unviable eggs), involving scientific practices of seeing and knowing about body parts, are brought together with the national politics of making borders and actively imagining nations. Thus this moment can be thought of as a "national imaginary," a moment when events and objects coalesce and at the same time enact the national borders.

Throughout this fieldnote, we have moments of measurement, registration, labeling and recording. Yet together with this there is yet another joke, about the patient's name. Whilst being anaesthetized and treated properly as a patient, her name is played upon with the reference to a "martyr" or suicide bomber, "shahid." Here we have biosociality and biopolitics: measuring and naming as unviable the eggs of the woman considered to be "other" to the nation, while reaffirming the practitioners' own status as dominant citizens.

"Transfer": eggs and the political "situation"

This third ethnographic account traces a twenty-four hour period during which resonances and ricochets in the discursive practices of ovum implantation and the political "situation" were particularly strong. This passage raises questions regarding what kinds of relations are being naturalized, and what kind of inversions of nature and culture are occurring.

Fieldnote

> The past 24 hours have been crazy. Yesterday evening just as I was riding the bus back to Jerusalem from Tel Aviv, a man blew himself up in the crowded "Beit-Israel" part of town. Nine people died. While I sat on the bus just as we were re-entering Jerusalem, I knew something was "up" because the driver increased the volume on the radio and everybody's mobile phones began to ring all around me. This is a sure sign that there had been a pigua[9], people hear about it on the news and call to check on loved ones to make sure they are safe. Indeed my own phone rang. It was Avram, my uncle, who told me about the explosion before I even had a chance to hear the radio announcer clearly.
>
> That night, at 4 a.m. I awoke to consecutive, loud booming sounds. These seemed to continue for quite a long time. I naively turned on the radio and television to see if there was any information on what was going on. They were reporting nothing. There was no siren to signal that I should go to the bomb shelter (which is a good thing because I did not know where this was!) so I stayed put. When morning came, the radio news reported that the IDF[10] had been bombing Bethlehem, just beyond the hills I could see from my study.
>
> In the morning I awoke and went to the hospital as usual, but with greater trepidation. At first I stayed in the clinic and observed the nurses talking to patients who came in with questions. They took phone calls from women wanting to know test results or about whether there were any eggs available for donation. After observing this for a while I went to the ward. Unusually, there was music playing in the laboratory which filtered into the surgery room. The physicians and nurses were talking politics with the laboratory technicians in the other room.
>
> On this day, there were three embryo transfers. To one patient, Biton said: "you might feel as though I am being aggressive but I want to remove as much of the *rir*, "mucous," as possible so that there are no obstructions to the embryo."[11] He then went into the laboratory to collect the embryos which the embryologists had prepared and left in a Petri dish for him under the microscope. He looked into the microscope and drew two embryos into the syringe. He then returned to the surgery room, where the embryos were inserted into the woman's vaginal canal and uterus.
>
> After observing the procedure Biton returned to his office and I with him. We talked between patient consultations about "the situation." Biton commented that, "it is very frightening here in Israel."[12]
>
> At home later that day after observing embryo transfer I turned on the television. The news program reported that a Palestinian man had opened fire at an Israeli military checkpoint and killed ten people. Next was an

interview with the father of one of the dead Israeli soldiers. He stated that his family are "proud Zionists" and that their son "died for the whole nation." The program began discussing the possibility of "transfer." This is shorthand, using the English word "transfer" and not the Hebrew word ha'avara. They meant, of course, "transferring" Palestinians from the Occupied Territories to somewhere else. One "option" discussed is "transferring" Palestinians in the West Bank to Gaza. The language is highly euphemistic. They were talking about ethnic cleansing. I wondered at how such a thing could be conceivable, occurring as it did less than sixty years after the holocaust. As I continued to watch television that evening with the news reporting "transfer" possibilities and a "martyred" Israeli man, I could not stop thinking about "embryo transfers" I had observed that day.

What is apparent here is that these are connections made by the researcher between two different kinds of transfer. Yet it is not simply that this connection was made because the two kinds of transfer were temporally juxtaposed in my research. Rather, metaphors of removal and implantation pervade both Israeli nationalistic discourses and IVF discourses. First, in the arena of nationalism, the history of expulsion of Palestinians from their lands in 1948 and present day expansion of settlements and Israeli borders within the West bank is a clear instance of this. Furthermore, since 1948 there has been the emergence of the social scientific disciplines of sociology and biblical archeology (among others) which in very practical ways created "proof" to justify nationalistic claims that Israel is a "land without a people for a people without a land" (Abu El Haj 1998, 2001; Dominguez 1989). This is one of the links between Israeli nationalism and other Euro-American imperialist projects.

Second, in the arena of the practices of Israeli ova extraction and exchange, my research has demonstrated Jewish-Israeli women rejecting ova from Palestinian-Israeli women (see Nahman 2006). Furthermore, the new law (which has not yet come into effect, but has been tabled in the Israeli Parliament) will make it illegal to donate ova between women of different religions. This has created limits of what can be transferred, and is another mode of ensuring that citizenship remains negotiable only through Jewish identity. Although these practices are not new in Israel, ova donation is one more route through which this kind of border gets made.

The language, so resonant, seemed actually to be referring to things which were worlds apart: "embryo transfer" for making babies, and the "transfer" referred to on the news about eliminating the enemy. This fieldnote, perhaps best illustrates the connections and naturalizations I am trying to examine in this essay. Not only are the two arenas of reproductive technologies and national belonging connected. They synecdochally co-produce one another. This connection between the part and the whole, as an "emic" kind of logic was apparent when the proud Jewish Israeli father asserted his son died for the nation. This kind of synecdochic, militarized logic is common to all kinds of nationalism. It is especially pertinent when it is juxtaposed with discussions of ethnic cleansing, euphemistically coded as "transfer."

Conclusion

It has been agreed by rabbis and inscribed in Israeli law that ova donation is permissible in Israel because of the Talmudic logic that gestation not genetics makes the kinship bond (see Kahn 2000 and Feldman and Wolowelsky 1997). This kind of naturalization of Jewish kinship is meant to promote the state's natality policies aimed at Jews and is one avenue of state management of the population. The legal and rabbinical ruling notwithstanding, for many of the Israelis I interviewed, IVF with egg donation means becoming a "natural" parent "artificially," as it is in most Euro-American contexts (Nahman 2006). There is an inversion of nature and culture where techniques of IVF are the mediators.

The disposability and transferability of ova through IVF has important gender dimensions. Not only are women's bodies the sites for this battle over citizenship and the national borders, but they are also the resource of "promissory capital" (Thompson 2005: 258). The future is being negotiated through knowledge, technology and promise, rather than solely through accumulation (ibid.). Ova extraction, exchange and implantation constitute sets of practices and discourses through which to see these rearticulations and reaffirmations of the relations between individuals and the state.

While the state of Israel was founded "artificially," this can be said of every state, and thus artificial inception is the natural way in which modern states arise. Crucially though, they arise through often violent extractions of people. This disposability of life can be seen both in the everyday practices along Israeli checkpoints and in clinics in discursive moments of construction of the national borders. Clearly these are different orders of exclusion and naturalization of the nation. But, I argue that these are fruitful couplings which demonstrate how biomedicine fits in to the consolidation of certain kinds of state power. Again, this is a kind of cyborg politics, which brings together different fragments or biosocial moments, and illustrates how they are fundamentally connected on various levels. Following Rabinow's work on the relationship between DNA and the collectivity, the way in which it is possible to know about the citizenship and collectivity in Israel are built into the techniques of ova extraction, exchange and implantation. This involves seeing the naturalization of a politics of "transfer" of Palestinians, and creation of borders and boundaries between Jewish and Israeli women in ova donation and the creation of national borders with walls and checkpoints; attention to the inherent violence in the naming practices of stabbing ovaries, and the globalized relations between research agendas of IVF units and relations between different national contexts. These relations are emblematic of biosociality. Feminist writings, which argue for an attention to the multiple and partial ways in which these connections get made help to extend the original conception of biosociality. Writing the synecdochal ways in which history, geography, capital get made, remade and undone in the micropractices of biomedicine facilitates a fertile ground for critique of national-state politics of expansion and consolidation.

Acknowledgments

This paper is based on research facilitated by the Wenner Gren Foundation for Anthropological Research and the Social Science and Humanities Research Council of Canada (SSHRC) (2000–2004). Several people have read through drafts of this paper and I want to thank them for their very helpful comments and suggestions. They are: Sahra Gibbon, Carlos Novas, Tiago Moreira, Maureen McNeil, Dave Weltman, Celia Roberts, Iris Jean-Klein, Bob Simpson, Lucy Suchman and Sarah Franklin.

Notes

1 Birman 2002, personal communication. Tzviya Birman is an Israeli social worker who specializes in egg and sperm donation.
2 Generally, this was the pattern of transnational ova donation in Israel. The clinic in which I conducted research, Global ART, was the first and only Israeli clinic to obtain Ministry of Health permission to import fertilized ova.
3 In Israel if one is of Mizrakhi ('Oriental') background, is a recent immigrant from the former Soviet Union or is an Arab, access to services and equality in treatment is not easily realizable unless one is more integrated into the middle classes (Dominguez 1989; Boyarin 1996; Lavie 1996).
4 This notion of Jewish survival is a complex and problematic one. On the one hand there are real historical reasons to have such concerns. On the other hand focusing solely on Jewish national survival ignores the historical periods and geographical locales in which survival, and integration within communities flourished (Shohat 2003).
5 'Legitimacy' is an important aspect of Israeli immigration. Not only is the 'quantity' of immigrants important, but the 'quality' of those immigrants is equally crucial (this is discussed in relation to ova donation in Nahman 2006).
6 This is a Jewish settlement on the West Bank.
7 A mashgikha is a woman from the Orthodox Jewish community who is employed to ensure that the practices adhere to Jewish rabbinical rules. See Kahn 2000 for an excellent discussion of this.
8 'Martyr' in Arabic. It is also another name for suicide bombers.
9 Pigua is the Hebrew word for 'attack'. But its root is the word 'injury', which connotes passivity. This is a perpetuation of the idea of the state of Israel as a 'victim' which can contribute to legitimizing its aggression.
10 Israeli Defense Forces.
11 In this sentence as is the case in many other medical and cultural contexts, the woman's own body is represented as an obstruction.
12 Biton and others commented to me that 'it is the worst time ever to be in Israel'. Interestingly, Jonathan Boyarin, writing in 1996 was told a similar thing by his interlocutors. In this case it would be fruitful to explore what kind of cultural work is being done by this notion of 'it's the worst time to be here'.

Bibliography

Abu El-Haj, N. (1998) "Translating truths: nationalism, the practice of archaeology, and the remaking of past and present in contemporary Jerusalem," *American Ethnologist*, 25: 166–88.

Abu El-Haj, N. (2001) *Facts on the Ground: Archaeological Practice and Territorial Self-Fashioning in Israeli Society.* Chicago, IL: University of Chicago Press.

Agamben, G. (1995) *Homo Sacer: Sovereign Power and Bare Life.* Stanford, CA: Stanford University Press.

Anderson, B. 1991 (1983) *Imagined Communities.* London and New York: Verso.

Boyarin J. 1996. *Palestine and Jewish History: Criticism at the Borders of Ethnography.* Minneapolis and London: University of Minneapolis Press.

Butler, J. (1993) *Bodies That Matter: On the Discursive Limits of "Se".* New York: Routledge.

Butler, J. (2004) *Precarious Life:The Powers of Mourning and Violence.* London: Verso.

Chernichovsky, D. (1992) "Health system reforms in industrialized democracies: an emerging paradigm," *The Millbank Quarterly*, 73.

Chernichovsky, D. and Chinitz, D. (1995) "The political economy of healthy system reform in Israel," *Health Economics*, 4: 127–41.

Dominguez, V. (1989) *People as Subject, People as Object: Selfhood and Peoplehood in Contemporary Israel.* Madison, WI: University of Wisconsin Press.

Douglas, M. (1966) *Purity and Danger: An Analysis of Pollution and Taboo.* London: Routledge.

Feldman, E. and Wolowelsky, J. B. (eds) (1997) *Jewish Law and the New Reproductive Technologies.* Hoboken, NJ: Ktav Publishing House.

Fielding, D. (2003) "How does civil war affect the magnitude of capital flight? Evidence from Israel during the Intifada." www.le.ac.uk/economics/research/RePEc/lec/leecon/dp03-10.pdf (accessed 03/02/05).

Foucault, M. (1978) *The History of Sexuality, Volume 1: An Introduction.* New York: Vintage Books.

Franklin, S. (1997) *Embodied Progress: A Cultural Account of Assisted Conception.* London: Routledge.

Franklin, S., Lury, C. and Stacey, J. (eds) (2000) *Global Nature, Global Culture.* London: Sage Publications.

Galili, L. (2005) "A Jewish demographic state," *Haaretz newspaper*, online. Israel.

Haraway, D. (1991) "A cyborg manifesto: science, technology, and socialist-feminism in the late twentieth century," *Simians, Cyborgs and Women: The Reinvention of Nature.* New York: Routledge.

Haraway, D. (1997) *Modest_Witness@ Second_Millenium. FemaleMan© Meets_Oncomouse™. Feminism and Technoscience.* New York: Routledge.

Hayden, C. P. (1995) "Gender, genetics and generation: reformulating biology in lesbian kinship," *Cultural Anthropology*, 10: 41–63.

Hubert, H. and Mauss, M. (1964) *Sacrifice: Its Nature and Function.* Chicago, IL: University of Chicago Press.

Ivry, T. (1999) "Reproduction as Martial Art." Paper presented at the annual conference of the International Institute of Sociology, Tel Aviv, Israel, June.

Kahn, S. M. (2000) *Reproducing Jews: A Cultural Account of Assisted Conception in Israel.* Durham, NC: Duke University Press.

Kanaaneh, R. (2002) *Birthing the Nation: Strategies of Palestinian Women in Israel.* Berkeley, CA: University of California Press.

Lavie S. 1996. "Blowups in the Borderzones: Third World Israelis Authors' Gropings for Home". In *Displacement, Diaspora and Geographies of Identity*, ed. S Lavie and T. Swedenburg. Durham, NC: Duke University Press

Levy, G. (2003) "She can go and give birth with Arafat," *Ha'aretz Newspaper* (Hebrew) 19 September.

Levy, G. (2006) "Neglected to death," *Ha'aretz Newspaper* (Hebrew) 16 January.

Mauss, M. (1990 [1950]) *The Gift: The Form and Reason for Exchange in Archaic Societies.* London: Routledge.

Nahman, M. (2006) "Materialising Israeliness: difference and mixture in transnational ova donation," *Science as Culture*, September.

Nahman, M. (forthcoming) "'The embryo method': an account of privatisation in transnational Israeli egg donation," in Birenbaum Carmeli, Daphna and Carmeli, Yoram S. (eds) *Kin, Gene, Community: Reproductive Technology among Jewish Israelis*, Oxford: Berghan Books.

Novas, C. and Rose, N. (2005) "Biological citizenship," in Ong, A. and Collier, S. J. (eds) *Global Assemblages: Technology, Politics, and Ethics as Anthropological Problems.* Malden, MA: Blackwell Publishing.

Portugese, J. (1998) *Fertility Policy in Israel: The Politics of Religion Gender and Nation.* London: Praeger Publishers.

Rabinerson, D., Dekel, A., Orvieto, R., Feldberg, D., Simon, D. and Kaplan, B. (2002) "Subsidised oocyte donation in Israel (1998–2000): results, costs and lessons," *Human Reproduction* 17: 1404–6.

Rabinow, P. (1995) "Artificiality and enlightenment: from sociobiology to biosociality," in *Essays in the Anthropology of Reason*. Princeton, NJ: Princeton University Press.

Rabinow, P. (1999) *French DNA: Trouble in Purgatory*. Chicago, IL: University of Chicago Press.

Shafir, G. (1999) "Zionism and colonialism: a comparative approach," in Pappé, I. (ed.) *The Israel/Palestine Question*. London: Routledge.

Shirom, A. (2001) "Private medical services in acute-care hospitals in Israel," *International Journal of Health Planning Management*, 16: 325–45.

Shohat, E. (2003) "Dislocated identities: reflections of an Arab Jew," in Kushner, T. and Solomon, A. (eds) *Wrestling With Zion: Progressive Jewish-American Responses to the Israeli-Palestinian Conflict*. New York: Grove Press.

Strathern, M. (1991) *Partial Connections.* Savage, MD: Rowman Littlefield.

Thompson, C. (2005) *Making Parents: The Ontological Choreography of Reproductive Technologies.* Cambridge, MA: MIT Press.

Titmuss, R. (1970) *The Gift Relationship*. London: Allen Unwin.

Verran, H. (1998) "Reimagining land ownership in Australia," *Postcolonial Studies*, 1: 237–54.

Yuval-Davis, N. (1989) "National reproduction and the 'demographic race' in Israel," in Yuval-Davis, N. and Anthias, F. (eds) *Woman-Nation-State*. London: Macmillan Press.

Yuval-Davis, N. (1997) *Gender and Nation*. London: Sage Publications.

7 Patients, profits and values

Myozyme as an exemplar of biosociality

Carlos Novas

Introduction: patients, profits and values

Since the birth of clinical medicine in the eighteenth century, the forms through which individuals are constituted as patients, the means by which revenues are generated from the treatment of illness, and the values invested in the promotion of the health and well-being of individuals and populations has undergone many changes. Today, I believe we are witnessing a transformation in the relationships between patients, profits and values. Paul Rabinow's (1996) essay, 'Artificiality and Enlightenment: From Sociobiology to Biosociality' provides a useful concept and some tools for investigating these transformations. In his essay, Rabinow was concerned with exploring the character of biopower today. One site where he chose to begin this investigation was the Human Genome Project (HGP) – a project that in 1992 was in its initial stages, and that has now been successfully completed. The HGP afforded Rabinow a site where he could begin to explore the 'practices of life' at 'one of the most potent present sites of new knowledges and powers'. Central to his reflections on biopower is its relation to modernity. By exploring biopower in relation to Foucault's discussion of the emergence of the modern epistemes of life (biology), labour (political economy), and language (philology) which contributed to the emergence of the figure of Man, Rabinow took up a theme that was never developed by Foucault due to his untimely death. Interestingly, Rabinow engages in dialogue with one of Foucault's contemporaries, Gilles Deleuze, to query whether the field of finitude characteristic of modern social formations has given way to a play of forces and forms which Deleuze has labelled the 'unlimited-finite' (Deleuze, 1988). The 'unlimited-finite' is a state in which beings have neither a perfected form, nor an essential opacity. According to Rabinow, the prime exponent of this state is DNA – an infinite number of beings have arisen from the four bases out of which DNA is constituted. In considering the possibilities created by the ability to know DNA in such a fashion that it is capable of being remade, Rabinow is concerned with interrogating novel practices emerging in the fields of life and labour which Deleuze claims could wash away the central figure of Man as the object and subject of knowledge characteristic of modernity. Rabinow is doubtful of some of Deleuze's epochal claims: his concerns are more limited and productive: he wants to investigate the significance of these novel practices by using the terms life, labour, and language heuristically.

I want to propose this reading of Rabinow's text throughout my paper. It is based on a reconsideration of the implications of what Rabinow means in his classic and rather cryptic proposition that '... in biosociality nature will be modelled on culture understood as practice. Nature will be known and remade through technique and will finally become artificial, just as culture becomes natural'. Given Rabinow's concerns in his essay to interrogate the limits of the modernist episteme and to question the nature/culture split, I think that what Rabinow is trying to get at here is how both nature and culture are comprised of a series of practices. I arrived at this formulation after finally making sense of his troubling (at least for me) statement: 'Practices make the person; or rather, they don't; they just make practitioners'. Rabinow made this statement in relation to Robert Castel's discussion of the distinction between disease and handicap. I believe that this distinction is central to understanding biosociality. Disease as a factor of risk requires isolation, quarantining and cure in order to prevent the contamination of the entire social body, whilst the notion of 'handicap' poses the question of what range of practices can be applied to a person or to the environment so that an individual can be made to perform a number of operations – in other words, to become a practitioner. Viewed through this lens, the problem that Rabinow is addressing in this essay and his ethnographic research in the field of the life sciences becomes intelligible in a new light. As he states 'My ethnographic question is: How will our social and ethical *practices* change as this project [the Human Genome Project] advances?' (my italics). He then qualifies this sentence by adding how he intends 'to approach this question on a number of levels and in a variety of sites'. I want to draw out some of the sociological implications of thinking of nature and culture as practice and the methodological lessons that can be drawn from Rabinow's approach to his ethnographic question. I want to concentrate on how attentiveness to the practices that go into making mouse models, developing business strategies, and crafting advertising campaigns makes it possible to consider some of the transformations that are taking place across the fields of life, labour, and language.

What I find useful about thinking through practices is that they provide a means of accounting for similarity and difference. As most introductory sociology textbooks tend to explain, despite the existence of great individual and group diversity, behaviour is nonetheless patterned in a regular fashion which produces enduring social forms that can be studied. Studying practices enables the analysis of similarity and difference whilst providing the room to manoeuvre between various levels of analysis – scale in a certain sense is accomplished through the assemblage of a range of practices. This approach draws attention to the past activities and present day actions that go into the assemblage of social relations and forms. I think what Rabinow is trying to do in 'Artificiality and Enlightenment' is to get us beyond starting with preconceived notions of what persons, nature, genetic advocacy groups, culture, firms, or the self are, and to inquire into how persons, nature, genetic advocacy groups, culture, firms, or the self are made up through a range of practices. This approach makes it possible to account for how certain practices and forms can continue over time and undergo change through the rearrangement of practices and the development of entirely new practices and forms. This approach further makes it possible to consider the movement of practices between different sites and forms. Practices developed to solve one problem may be applicable to those that emerge at another time and place to create a new configuration or assemblage. This makes it possible to consider how both the old and the new can quite comfortably sit side by side, or just as equally grate against one another.

Let me put this another way by using the example of biotechnology firms. They all similarly engage in a range of activities that are oriented towards raising capital, generating economic value, protecting their intellectual property assets, and marketing their products. However, each biotechnology firm is slightly different from one another based on their staff, products, markets, competitors and so on. Depending on the ways that a small number of practices are sutured together, they can produce great diversity in terms of the form that a biotechnology company takes. The scale at which a biotechnology firm is able to operate is dependent on its abilities to coordinate a range of practices at a number of different sites. Indeed, there are specialist practitioners whose task it is to do this work of co-ordinating practices. These types of practitioners are variously called managers, directors, CEOs and in some cases, presidents. To a certain extent, differences between individuals or firms can be partially accounted for in terms of how they assemble together a range of practices. Thinking about biotechnology firms as an assemblage of practices that are material, cultural and intellectual in scope makes it possible to consider how lay persons can become involved in the scientific research of a biotechnology company. In a certain sense they become scientific practitioners. As we know from the work of Bruno Latour (1987), science involves a considerable range of activities that extends beyond wearing a white coat and working in a laboratory. Lay individuals and groups can become scientific practitioners when they help to raise funds for biomedical research, facilitate the collection of blood and tissue samples, collect and share data about a disease, shape legislation relating to scientific research, or provide scientific or medical information to their membership and physicians.

However, not everyone has equal access to the resources that are required to put social practices in motion or to becoming a practitioner. In the case of medicine, there are very good reasons for not allowing everyone to practise this art, but at the same time, the persons who are presently authorised to be medical practitioners are a product and outcome of a protracted historical struggle. Thinking about inequality in relation to practices makes it possible to consider how despite the uneven distribution of access to resources, individuals, social groups and corporations can sometimes skilfully use, develop and assemble together a range of practices that can both challenge and overcome differences in size, scale and power. Furthermore, it becomes possible to begin to think about how individuals and collectives can become skilled at using particular practices even if they have no formal training in their use. As most of us are aware, social practices can also be dividing: they can be used to exclude just as much as they can be used to include. The discourses and practices we deploy in relation to categories such as gender, race, ethnicity, illness, personhood, and citizenship affects the ways we treat persons, the resources they are given access to, and how they are able to conduct their lives.

Paying attention to practices also lets us focus on how people attempt to build particular futures. It concentrates attention on the present day range of activities and forms of thought that individuals and collectives use to shape the character of practices, routines, forms, institutions, firms, nature and culture in the future (Brown, 2003; Brown *et al.*, 2000; Hedgecoe and Martin, 2003; Shostak, 2004). The same could be said of the past. The past has been made up and is being made up in the present by a whole range of practices. In considering biosociality, I am interested in the analysis of who has the power to create particular futures, how those futures are made, and who is excluded from these visions of the future. Similar to Rabinow, I share a concern with investigating how our social and ethical practices are changing as a result of the possibilities created through the capacity to know and intervene upon life in such a fashion that it is capable of being remade. My present research concentrates on the hopes and expectations that are invested by a selective range of patients' organisations and biotechnology firms in the development of cures and treatments. This dyad provides ample opportunities to explore the similar, yet different range of practices through which biotechnology firms and patient's groups transform life into a resource for the generation of health and wealth (Novas, 2006; Waldby, 2000, 2002). As part of the exploration of this field, I am committed to analysing how developments in the field of law, capital markets, manufacturing technologies, information technologies, branding and science interact with one another.

This is a very roundabout way of getting to the argument I want to develop in my paper. In exploring the character of biosociality, I want to avoid restricting it exclusively to the realm of patients' groups as so many sociological and anthropological accounts have done. What I will do is concentrate on the different, yet similar range of practices employed by patients' groups and biotechnology firms to develop cures or therapies in order to explore the affinities between them. Second, using this dyad as a guide, I will draw upon my current research which focuses on the range of practices through which biotechnology firms and patient organisations are involved in the production of biomedical futures. This dyad provides ample opportunities to explore the forms and modalities through which these types of organisations attempt to create and embed particular visions of the future in biological organisms, in economies for the production and distribution of health, and in the discourses of ethics and marketing. One site of my current empirical investigations is the biotechnology firm Genzyme. What interested me in this firm are its efforts to communicate and engage in dialogue with patients' organisations. As part of studying Genzyme's efforts to develop a treatment for Pompe disease, I have concentrated on its partnerships with university researchers and the firms it has acquired. In this paper, I will focus on one firm acquired by Genzyme, Novazyme. Novazyme is interesting since its chief executive officer

(CEO), John Crowley, has two children affected by Pompe disease. Prior to his leadership of Novazyme, Crowley had established a disease advocacy group known as the Children's Pompe Foundation. This firm provides a useful case study by which to think about contemporary biopolitics by examining the relationships between hope, capitalism and the life sciences. I will then move on to discuss the range of practices through which Genzyme has developed a treatment for Pompe disease known as Myozyme. The development of this treatment provides a means of examining the intersection between the life sciences, political economy, and language.

John Crowley, Novazyme and entrepreneurial salvation

Within the sociological and anthropological literature, biosociality is often referenced to indicate the growing involvement of patients and lay persons in scientific research (Heath, 1998; Rapp, 2000, 2003; Rose and Novas, 2005) The participation of patients and their carers in research reflects the prominence of science as a place where hopes for therapies or cures are invested and is indicative of how we are driven to seek to overcome our biological fates through the application of even more technoscience. The growing participation of patients and lay persons in science can be seen as part of the reformulation of the interrelated problems of how we should treat and care for the sick and infirm individuals and at the same time promote the health of the population. Increasing patient and lay participation in science is indicative of growing dissatisfaction with the medical profession and scientists for the ways in which they attempt to manage health on an individual and collective basis. Paradoxically, it is also an expression of confidence in the ability of the medical and scientific establishment to act upon the health of each and all of us and to develop novel cures or therapies provided that it is able to incorporate the demands, experiences and insights of non-scientists. This raises questions about the kinds of contributions that non-scientists make to medicine and scientific research. The one, but by no means exclusive contribution that I want to focus attention on is the range of practices that are managerial in orientation through which patients, carers, and patients' groups become involved in the management of scientific research activities in the hopes of accelerating the development of therapies or cures.

To highlight some of the ways non-scientists have become involved in the creation and management of biomedical futures, I will focus on the experience of John and Aileen Crowley, who have two children affected by Pompe disease. In response to this illness, the Crowleys established a patients' group dedicated to funding research on this disease. John's experience as a business strategist for Bristol Myers Squib, combined with his training as a Harvard MBA graduate led him to take up a position as the CEO of a biotechnology company that was developing a therapy for his children's illness. The highly atypical and unrepresentative character of their experiences makes it useful for analysing some of the practices that individuals and patients' organisations are assembling together in order to help realise the potential of the new genetics to develop therapies or cures. The way that I will approach the experiences of the Crowleys is by concentrating on two forms through which they were mediated in the press: the human interest story and the corporate press release. The narrative forms and content of these media genres provide an interesting locale by which to explore the intersection between hope, science and capitalism that form part of the reconfiguration of the relations between life, labour and language. It further provides the opportunity to critically explore lay participation in scientific research, the affinities between the practices employed by patients' organisations and biotechnology firms, and the centrality of managerial practices to the realisation of the kinds of futures created by these types of organisations.

The human interest story constitutes one of the dominant representational practices through which the press discusses promissory scientific and therapeutic futures (Henderson and Kitzinger, 1999; Petersen, 2001). These types of stories concisely suture together personal illness experiences, lay and professional attempts to raise awareness of specific diseases, and discussions of the social, ethical and economic consequences of the march of scientific progress. In the case of John and Aileen Crowley, their experiences have featured on the front page of the *Wall Street Journal*, the magazine pages of *Exceptional Parent*, a Harvard Business School case study, and in a number of radio and television programmes. A book has been written about their experiences and the possibility exists for a film to be produced about them featuring the actor Harrison Ford (Anand, 2006). As a media narrative, the Crowley story is a tale about American heroism (Hughes, 1968). Heroic tales, I believe, can tell us something about the kinds of behaviour, forms of sociality, and objects that are culturally valued at a particular historical moment.

Reading these kinds of stories, it's hard not to be emotionally affected by the suffering experienced by the Crowleys' children and to admire John and Aileen's efforts to develop a cure for their disease. Megan and Patrick, as the media explain, were diagnosed with a rare, terminal illness within the first year of their life. Doctors did not expect them to live beyond the age of two.[1] They are also dependent on nursing care 24 hours a day, rely on ventilators to help them breathe, and are fed through gastrointestinal tubes. Patrick and Aileen Crowley have gone to considerable lengths and expense to keep their children alive and well. John further took the extraordinary step of becoming the CEO of a biotechnology firm to develop a cure for his children's illness. Empathy, compassion, and hope: these are the kinds of feelings human interest stories are crafted to evoke (Hughes, 1968). In many of the stories I studied, these feelings were evoked through drawing upon two tropes that were also used to account for John's extraordinary efforts, dedication and sense of urgency. These tropes involved the use of temporal metaphors such as how 'time is running out' or the 'clock is ticking' against Megan and Patrick. Second, John Crowley's efforts to 'save his children' was routinely described as a 'quest' or 'crusade' due to his extraordinary effort to quickly develop a cure for them. As a media narrative, this is a thoroughly modern tale: religious metaphors intersect with the presentation of science as means to deliver us from our ills and the acceleration of the pace of scientific progress through the application of even more knowledge and industry is considered to be a rational and worthwhile endeavour.

The forms through which the Crowleys' experiences were framed and narrated by the media in terms of a 'quest' or 'crusade' to 'save their children' tells us a great deal about the kinds of behaviour, work ethos, response to illness, and forms of sociality that are valorised in the contemporary American press (Hughes, 1968). In the case of John Crowley, his quest began immediately after Megan's diagnosis in March 1998. John began consulting the Internet to learn more about the disease. Shortly afterwards, he began to contact and meet scientists. In August 1998, John and Aileen founded the Children's Pompe Foundation to raise money to accelerate research efforts that could lead to a cure. In little over a year, this organisation raised $1.2 million towards this end. This foundation funded the research of the principal laboratories in the United States conducting research on Pompe disease. The one scientist who the media focused attention upon in their stories was Dr William Canfield. Whilst at the University of Oklahoma, Canfield developed a novel method of producing therapeutic enzymes. He eventually founded a biotechnology company called Targeted Therapy in 1999. Like many biotech start-up companies, Canfield had difficulty attracting venture capital and a chief executive officer. He proposed that Crowley, a Harvard MBA graduate, should run the company. After carefully considering it for some time, in March 2001 Crowley quit his job as a business strategist at Bristol Myers Squib, borrowed $100,000 against his home and retirement plan, and became CEO of Targeted Therapy which he renamed Novazyme. As most of the press stories narrate, this move allowed John Crowley to dedicate all of his time to finding as quickly as possible a cure for his children's illness.

Media accounts of John Crowley celebrate the American entrepreneurial spirit. These stories not only locate hopes for cures or treatments in science, but in the spirit of capitalism. These stories highlight a work ethic and a form of devotedness characteristic of contemporary American corporate culture. In attempting to save his children, the press valorise John's immediate efforts to learn more about Megan's and Patrick's illness by consulting the Internet, waking up early to keep abreast of research developments, zigzagging across the United States and Europe to speak to scientists, and after a day at work, staying up late planning fundraising events for the Children's Pompe Foundation (D'Aurizio, 1999a, 1999b). As a narrative of American entrepreneurial heroism, the moral message of these tales suggests that the best way to devote yourself to the enterprise of saving your children is through becoming knowledgeable about their illness and by becoming actively involved in seeking to develop a cure. What these stories fail to communicate, is the sense of fear, worry, frustration, anxiety and distress experienced by John and Aileen Crowley, alongside their children, Megan and Patrick as they have had to encounter a terminal illness (the only articles which discussed these aspects appeared in *Exceptional Parent*, 2000a, 2000b).

This ethos of work and dedication being described by the media in relation to Crowley figures prominently in American managerial corporate culture. Central to this ethos is the discipline of working upon oneself in a continuous fashion so as to produce an efficient, adaptable and enterprising subject who is able to cope with a range of personal, economic and social exigencies (Deleuze, 1995). The narration of the Crowley story by the media suggests that this kind of work ethic should inform how individuals respond to illness. Individuals should not only play an active role alongside doctors in providing for their own health and that of their families, but they must also play an active role in helping to develop therapies or treatments that will cure. Although the example of John Crowley is extreme and unique, the narration of his story by the media generally serves to valorise the kinds of behaviour and forms of sociality that are esteemed in states where neoliberal rationalities of government encourage the infusion of the spirit of capitalism in all social relations. By using the experience of John Crowley, the media suggest that the infusion of a corporate ethos into the organisation of patients' groups that are oriented towards the development of cures or therapies can reduce the horizons of scientific hopes. By celebrating the American managerial and entrepreneurial spirit, media stories relating to John Crowley further champion the market as a site where things can get done quickly and efficiently. Central to this spirit is the conquest of nature and time: both of which require massive amounts of funds.[2] The investment of capital is required to develop therapies which act upon the biological pathways of a disease and alter its natural developmental time scale. In championing John Crowley's leadership of a biotechnology firm, the press celebrates the partnership between science and capitalism as the most efficient means of providing for the health and well-being of individuals and populations. At the very least, what this suggests is that the press plays an important role in shaping the contours of biosociality and contemporary identity practices in relation to new biomedical knowledges and technologies.

Corporate press releases provide a different insight into the relationship between science capitalism and therapeutic futures. Just like human interest stories, the accounts that corporate press releases provide are always partial in that they are statements designed to communicate a particular narrative of the firm. Using the example of Novazyme, I want to concentrate on how firms use press releases to communicate how they are managing the scientific and therapeutic futures embodied in their research activities and the products they are developing.

Although the content of Novazyme's press releases vary, a story that was consistently told by this firm was that it is a biotechnology company which uses its 'proprietary phosphorylation technologies in the search for effective biotherapies for the fifty known lysosomal storage diseases that afflict humans. Novazyme will capitalize on its depth of scientific, research and managerial expertise to rapidly develop novel enzyme replacement therapies in this area' (PR Newswire, 2000). The features of this statement that I would like to concentrate on are proprietary technologies, phosphorylation, lysosomal storage diseases, enzyme replacement therapies and capitalisation. The proprietary technologies referred to were developed by Dr William Canfield. He developed a novel method of producing therapeutic enzymes by developing a recombinant Chinese Hamster Ovary (CHO) cell line that produced highly phosphorylated human enzymes. Canfield's advance consisted of a unique method of attaching a mannose-6 phosphate to enzymes which help lysosomes within the cell recognise it as if it was naturally produced by the body. This innovation was claimed to potentially lead to the development of more effective biotherapies for a group of diseases which are known as lysosomal storage disorders. This group of over fifty diseases are thought to be caused by a malfunction in the body's capacity to produce a specific enzyme which results in the accumulation of glycogen in the lysosomes of cells. These disorders can be treated by replacing the missing enzyme. This is what is meant by the term enzyme replacement therapy (ERT). According to Novazyme, it was claimed that existing forms of ERT rely on flooding a patient's body with the enzyme in the hope that it will eventually be taken up by cells. By way of contrast, Novazyme's methods of producing ERT by targeting specific cell receptors reduces dosage rates and was claimed to increase the efficaciousness of ERT, thereby minimising the potential for side effects. Novazyme presented itself as an organisation dedicated to developing biotherapies for all lysosomal storage disorders – a market estimated to be worth $5 billion.[3] Novazyme's ability to generate revenue from this market by developing ERT which enhances the health of persons affected by LSD required it to capitalise on its scientific research and managerial expertise. In claiming the potential for this firm to become a leader in this sector, John Crowley expressed confidence 'that with the scientific and managerial expertise that we currently have at Novazyme, we will be able to achieve this goal in a timely manner' (PR Newswire, 2000). What I believe is of relevance from Novazyme's press releases is the emphasis on the combination of good science, effective management, and a sense of timeliness as being essential ingredients to the generation of value from its capitalisation in the therapeutic futures of LSD and ERT.

   Press releases tell us about the kinds of images firms want to project about themselves and the kinds of practices that they consider essential to securing the continued commitment of the diverse range of actors who invest in corporate futures (which can be seen from Novazyme's press releases chronologically). The story communicated by this firm over time was its rapid progression and effective management on a number of fronts. This ranged from obtaining start-up funds from angel investors, raising $8 million in Series A private equity financing (subsequently $16 million), gaining Orphan Drug designation for Pompe disease and mucopolysaccharidosis (MPS 1), building the manufacturing capacity to produce recombinant enzymes, demonstrating the efficaciousness of their experimental therapy in a mouse model study, to considering conducting human clinical trials. The press releases communicate a developmental pathway essential to securing the commitment of venture capitalists – a sound scientific platform and management plan which ensures the rapid movement of a therapy from the laboratory to the clinic. The faster this motion takes place, the quicker a rate of return is realised on the capital and hope invested. This motion was completed in August 2001 when Novazyme was acquired by Genzyme for $137.5 million. This deal included the possibility of an additional $87.5 million payout contingent on marketing approval for two products developed with Novazyme's technology. The profitable expectations of the venture capitalists who invested in the promissory futures of Novazyme were satisfied – many of them realised a six-fold return on their investment (Anand, 2003). As part of this deal, John Crowley was appointed as Vice President of Genzyme Therapeutics – a position which included responsibility for its Pompe programme. As for the hopes of patients especially those affected by Pompe disease who invested in Novazyme's promissory futures, these effectively became monopolised by Genzyme, the only firm working on a therapy for their illness.

By concentrating on how experiences of the Crowleys and Novazyme were mediated, these stories tell us about the centrality of contemporary managerial discourses and practices that help to shape how individuals, patients' groups and corporations go about the enterprise of creating biomedical futures. The example of John Crowley brings into focus the highly similar practices of administrating a patient's organisation and directing a biotechnology firm (cf. Couzin, 2005). In this highly untypical and unrepresentative case, at the leadership level, the two are fused together.[4] As a heuristic device, this case can teach some important lessons about the intersections between hope, science and capitalism. First, the distinctions between the practices employed by patients' organisations and biotechnology firms are not as clear cut as commonly supposed. The sets of skills which John employed to raise funds for the Children's Pompe Foundation in order to create a future cure for the disease can be put to use in equally good measure in mobilising venture capitalists to invest in the biomedical futures crafted by Novazyme. The homologies between these sets of practices are rooted in contemporary organisational and bureaucratic cultures. The difference between them is solely a matter of scale and purpose: to accomplish the development of cures or therapies, one set of practices relies upon the management and mobilisation of altruism, whilst the other relies upon the management of the promise of generating profitable returns or dividends. The second lesson that can be drawn from this case study is that we need to broaden our conceptions of what science is and how patients or lay persons contribute to it. As many studies in the field of STS indicate, science consists of a broader range of activities than working at a lab bench. In the case of the biotechnology industry, it requires good management and scientific practices. Although John does not have any formal qualifications as a scientist, he *is* a scientific practitioner: he became competent at understanding the scientific and medical literature related to his children's condition, organising a group of patients, carers and benefactors to raise funds to support research efforts aimed at quickly developing a cure, successfully managing the development of Novazyme and ensuring that its scientific practices were infused with capital. Lastly, the Crowley story indicates the need to be cautious about the celebratory tone of media and academic discussions of lay involvement in science. In studying patients' organisations, more attention needs to be focused on the specific racial, gendered and socio-material bases on which particular individuals and groups get to create biomedical futures.

As the media narrated the experiences of the Crowleys, they helped to reinforce a gendered division of labour when it comes to caring for sick and infirm children. A large proportion of the press stories that relate to the Crowley family rarely make any reference to Aileen. She is generally portrayed as the devoted wife and mother who supports John and looks after the kids while he busily and devotedly endeavours to save his children. No credit was given to Aileen in the press for her work to help develop a cure for Pompe disease. It is also important to emphasise how access to the practices and resources required to create biomedical futures are unevenly distributed along the lines of race, gender and social class. The infusion of a corporate ethos into patients' groups is no doubt a result of the leadership and membership of these groups being increasingly drawn from the professional sector (Savage, 2005). The Crowley story is instructive here: many of the newspapers articles downplay the fact that John is a lawyer and a Harvard MBA graduate. Alternatively, they tend to emphasise how a man with only a high school background in biology not only established a charitable foundation, but also become the CEO of a firm dedicated to finding a cure for his children's illness. A large proportion of the press stories concentrated on the childhood form of the illness and only a few mentioned how it could also manifest itself in adults. Childhood sufferers of illnesses have greater access to the representational and social resources required to influence the future of their disease, often to the exclusion or detriment of adult sufferers (Beard, 2004; Stockdale, 1999; Stockdale and Terry, 2002). Lastly, like many genetic advocacy groups founded in the wake of the Human Genome Project, they tend to place an overarching organisational emphasis on funding scientific research (Terry, 2003). Whilst in the past patients' groups were oriented toward providing support and a kind of welfare benefit to individuals and families to help them cope with their condition, contemporary patients' organisations are more focused on providing financial and managerial assistance to the medical and scientific establishment in the hopes that it will lead to the more rapid development of cures or therapies.

The John Crowley story provides a means of thinking through the novel sites and experiences where scientific devotedness is practised and how the languages of salvation, philanthropy and entrepreneurialism are being contemporaneously reconfigured, shaping the contours of biosociality in America. This story is indicative of the pathways that have been created between citizens, the life sciences, market forces, and the media. I want to follow the Novazyme pathway to see where it leads – at the present moment, it most obviously takes me to Genzyme.

Genzyme, orphan diseases, and medical markets

In his essay, Paul Rabinow was concerned with exploring how the emergence of novel practices in the life sciences could give rise to changes in the fields of labour and language. Using the example of Genzyme and its development of a treatment for Pompe disease, I want to explore how Genzyme is involved in the artifice of remaking life, creating markets for orphan disease treatments, and using language and signs to brand its products. This makes it possible to consider the various ways in which this firm makes up nature, therapies, markets, value, norms, Genzyme, identities, consumers and social orders through a diverse range of practices. By thinking about the practices through which this firm developed

Myozyme, it provides a means of exploring some of the transformations that have taken place across the fields of life, labour, and language.

Genzyme was founded in 1981. It was one firm amongst the many that were created shortly after the establishment of the safety of recombining DNA from different species. Whilst the novel practices emerging in the life sciences no doubt gave birth to scores of enterprises such as Genzyme, one medium that fostered the development of the biotechnology industry was a series of legislative and legal reforms that took place in the United States in the early 1980s. The passage of the Bayh-Dole Act (1980) created novel inducements to commercialise academic research. The reform of the patent system through the Patent and Trademark Amendment Act (1980) combined with expansion of the boundaries of patentability to include biotechnological inventions through the landmark Supreme Court decision in Charkrabarty v. Diamond contributed to the further growth of this industry. Lastly, the Orphan Drug Act (1983) created the appropriate legal and market incentives to channel firms such as Genzyme into pathways conducive to the development of treatments for rare diseases (Ashton, 2001; Haffner, 2003; Haffner *et al.*, 2002). Of course, from the 1980s onwards the form and character of biotechnology firms have undergone considerable transformation – no doubt brought about as a result of the development of even more novel practices in the life sciences, the growing availability of public equity, the creation of specialised financial markets, tax incentives, and national strategies to promote the development of the biotechnology industry. To understand the novel bonds that are being formed across the fields of life and labour, we need to pay attention to the range of practices that have assembled, shaped and given form to contemporary biotechnology firms. This makes it possible to consider how biotechnology firms are involved in a continuous process of unfolding or becoming through their day-to-day activities and how they are involved in remaking nature and culture.

Although all biotechnology firms differ from one another, Genzyme is considered by many analysts to be unique (Robbins-Roth, 2000). How is Genzyme different? Under the leadership of Henri Termeer from 1983 onwards, Genzyme has been committed to ensuring that it was more than simply a firm that sold its ideas to pharmaceutical companies. Second, Genzyme specialises in 'diseases and conditions with unmet medical needs'. Its focus on rare conditions such as Pompe disease is due to the success it has had with a treatment for Gaucher's disease; a rare lysosomal storage disorder which affects approximately 3,000–5,000 individuals worldwide. By developing Ceredase in 1991, Genzyme provided 'proof of concept' that enzyme replacement therapy (ERT) could be used to effectively treat a LSD. To overcome problems associated with the production of Ceredase,[5] Genzyme developed a recombinant version known as Cerezyme in 1994. Third, as sales of these therapies accounted for over 60 per cent of Genzyme's annual revenues, it provided 'proof of principle' that you could efficaciously make up a significant market out of a small patient population (Office of Technology Assessment, 1992). Firms such as Novazyme tried to capitalise on these novel market possibilities. To continue its leadership in this field, Genzyme has developed therapies and markets in Fabry's disease, MPS 1, and Pompe disease. I want to focus on the development of Myozyme since it enables me to draw attention to the practices and scale that give form to Genzyme. These practices range in scale from the molecular level, to the organisation and branding of this firm, the dynamics of the orphan drug industry, and global biopolitics.

Biotechnology firms such as Genzyme harness the capacity to intervene upon DNA to create useful products and services that contain the potential to generate economic revenue. Using the example of Myozyme, I want to illustrate two forms through which this corporation is involved in the artifice of making up nature or biology. First, Genzyme is involved in the production of nature through genetically engineering Chinese Hamster Ovary (CHO) cell lines to produce human acid alpha-glucocidase. The biology of these cells is thus modified to fulfil therapeutic objectives and live in an industrial environment. To enable recombinant CHO cells to excrete human enzymes, they are progressively cultured in larger and larger stainless steel vats known as bioreactors. Bioreactors contain the appropriate nutrient medium and temperature for recombinant cells to thrive in a specially designed artificial environment that complies with medico-industrial manufacturing norms and practices.[6] The development of recombinant CHO cell lines and their cultivation in bioreactors requires considerable expertise, artifice and capital. A second form through which Genzyme remakes life is by acting upon the pathological processes associated with Pompe disease. Myozyme, like all therapeutic interventions upon the body is concerned with altering the biological pathways and timescale of the manifestation of disease so that it is in accordance with culturally bound conceptions of human health and lifespan. The lives of persons affected by Pompe disease will be artificially sustained by Myozyme; a therapeutic enzyme produced by recombinant CHO cells which mimics the action of naturally occurring human acid alpha-glucosidase. The development of Myozyme illustrates how the fusion of industrial-entrepreneurial settings with the novel techniques that have emerged in the life sciences can result in the creation of novel conditions for the existence of humans and CHO cells. This is what biosociality is about: the blurring of the boundaries between nature and culture and the folding of the fields of life, labour and language into new configurations.

What is significant about the emergence of biotechnology firms such as Genzyme is that they successfully merge together the life sciences, capital and the pursuit of profit. As a firm, Genzyme is composed though the combination of value generating practices and the practices through which it articulates its corporate identity and moral values. Genzyme is dependent on its ability to raise capital and generate revenue from the development of therapies such as Myozyme. Its capacity to develop therapies in the present is a product of its past organisational decisions and capitalisation structures. In terms of its past capitalisation structure, Genzyme was a pioneer in the use of tracking stocks. Tracking stocks are thought to enable a firm to raise more capital, in contrast to conventional means of raising finance, by dividing a firm into different divisions. This enables investors to 'unlock' the value present in the different avenues of research that a firm is pursuing which may have gone unnoticed by investors if it was simply included under the umbrella of a large corporation. Despite the division of a firm into multiple entities, tracking stocks enable a company to have a single board of directors, offset losses in one division against its overall taxation burden, share resources, intellectual property and personnel across divisions at cost price, rather than market price (Salter and Green, 2001). Although this capitalisation strategy was successful, Genzyme abandoned tracking stocks in 2003 since it no longer fit into its business objectives (Watson, 2003). Second, the successful development of ERT such as Ceredase and Cerezyme, combined with some of its other successful products and services have provided Genzyme with the sources of revenue required to sustain its research programmes and the commitment of investors. Third, Genzyme's mergers and acquisition policy over a number of years have enabled it to develop the proprietary technologies, manufacturing capacity and expertise to develop novel therapeutic agents, not only in the case of Pompe disease, but also across all its fields of research. Lastly, Genzyme's commitment to building a vertically integrated firm since its inception have allowed it to retain the economic, intellectual and human resource value generated at all stages of the drug development process – from the lab bench to marketing. In comparison with other biotechnology firms, Genzyme has a unique and diversified corporate structure – and one that is profitable.

Myozyme is not only an enzyme designed through the techniques of recombinatorial genetics: it also helps to realise and bear the values of the firm that brought it into being. Therapies such as Myozyme not only generate revenue streams, they also bear the moral and social values of the firms that bring them into being. Genzyme is not simply a firm, but a brand in and of itself. Central to the construction of this brand is a commitment to developing treatments for 'diseases and conditions with unmet medical needs' (see www.genzyme.com). Genzyme manifests its corporate values, civility and identity through a number of practices: the construction of its corporate headquarters as one of the most environmentally friendly buildings in the United States, the provision of Ceredase and Cerezyme free of cost to Gaucher's patients in a number of developing countries, and its commitment to interacting with stakeholders such as genetic advocacy groups. It further enacts itself as a benevolent corporate entity by providing a range of services to patients and their families. These services include genetic counselling, information on a disease and its forms of treatment, insurance advice, and disease specific websites such as www.pompe.com. These types of services display considerable overlap with those offered by patients' organisations. A key difference, however, is their orientation towards generating economic value by developing Genzyme's branded identity. For example, the www.pompe.com website is a comprehensive online resource Genzyme created for the Pompe community. It is also a site for developing meaningful relationships with 'customers' through an 'online education strategy' which not only provides meaningful information, but also adds value to this firm's bottom lines (PR Newswire, 2003). The realisation of value from Genzyme's branded identity relies jointly upon the construction of this firm as benevolent social actor and as an organisation that can develop therapies for persons whose medical needs are presently unmet.

Myozyme forms part of Genzyme's business strategy to build markets for diseases whose needs are presently unmet. Much like Ceredase, Cerezyme and Fabryzyme, Myozyme is expected to generate substantial revenues for this firm despite the fact that Pompe disease affects less than 10,000 individuals worldwide. Myozyme, on a broader scale of analysis contributes to the formation of the political economies that make possible orphan disease markets. Without doubt, the existence of these political economies is made possible through the tax incentives and monopoly provisions contained in the United States Orphan Drug Act and the European Orphan Medicinal Products regulations. This legislation espouses the principle that the market can be used as a mechanism to correct a market failure and at the same time accomplish the socially and economically desirable objective of developing cures or therapies for populations affected by rare diseases. Genzyme's first economically successful therapy, Ceredase, is in many ways a product of this legislation. However, Ceredase not only validated Genzyme's unusual business strategy, it helped to promote a novel logic of accumulation into the biotechnology and pharmaceutical industries. Ceredase, and now Myozyme challenge the conventional economic logics present in these industries. They counter the principle that the market fails to develop treatments for diseases which affect a small patient population since firms will not be able to recuperate their research and development expenses. Genzyme's business strategy provides a profitable example that the market can be used to correct one of its shortcomings and at the same time provide benefits to medically marginalised populations.

What is significant about Genzyme's contributions to the accumulation logic of orphan drug political economies is that its pricing practices fold the costs of being kept alive through medical treatment into a new configuration. Genzyme's strategy has consisted of targeting diseases that impose a heavy personal medical burden and incur high hospitalisation costs. For example, the annual medical costs of treating a child affected by Pompe disease runs into the region of $250,000. As ERT often restores bodily function and sometimes reverses the effects of a disease, they can command a high price. The annual costs of treating a patient with Myozyme are estimated to be in the region of $70,000 to $250,000 dependent on dosage and body weight. This pricing structure represents significant savings for national health systems and private insurance providers, a better quality of life for patients, and a significant source of corporate revenue since ERT are required throughout a patient's lifetime. Of course, this pricing strategy rests on getting paid. Here, Genzyme's contribution to orphan drug political economies is highly interesting: it works with national health authorities, private insurance companies and patients' groups to ensure that the therapies it has developed are reimbursed. Through practices ranging from the development of therapies by inserting human DNA into CHO cell lines to creating orphan drug political economies, Genzyme's corporate activities help to give form and shape to contemporary biopolitics.

Whilst biopolitics in the past was bound up with nations and states, it contemporaneously takes place on a global scale. Genzyme indicates how generating revenue from satisfying unmet medical needs is a truly global enterprise – at least global in reach to the markets that can diagnose these illnesses and treat them: predominantly North America, Europe and Australasia. The creation of orphan disease political economies begs questions about how the individual and collective welfare needs of this population are administered. In allocating responsibility for the development of treatments for orphan diseases to the market, the state allocates some of its powers over life to biotechnology and pharmaceutical companies. Increasingly, corporations such as Genzyme are the only ones who can provide for the health and well being of individuals and populations affected by rare diseases. For persons affected by Pompe disease, Genzyme is their only hope. This raises questions about the political economy underpinning the creation of markets in unmet medical needs. Although the dynamics of these economies are novel, the use of market solutions to achieve social objectives is troubled by a problem that has beleaguered economic theory since the eighteenth century: the market only offers its luxuries to those that can afford them. In the United States, access to medical care and therapies such as Myozyme are stratified along racial and social lines. Furthermore, these exclusionary practices intersect with a global politics of life and death. This form of politics sees the vitality of children from affluent nations enhanced through expensive and life-long treatments, whilst those from poorer nations are left to die for lack of treatment of common ailments such as diarrhoea. Practices, it seems, play a role in deciding who lives and who dies.

Conclusion

Paul Rabinow's essay invites readers to question the limits of modern social formations. In considering how the Human Genome Project would affect our social and ethical practices, Rabinow was concerned with exploring how the fields of life, labour and language which Michel Foucault considered essential to the formation of modernity were undergoing a process of transformation. Similar to Michel Foucault's, *The Birth of the Clinic*, I believe that Rabinow's brief essay attempts to teach a methodological lesson. His discussion of transformations in the concept of risk, the distinction between disease and disability, changes in agricultural production, boutique tomatoes, and cryptic passages from Rimbaud are oriented towards focusing our attention on how transformations to the character of modern social formations takes place along a number of seemingly unconnected sites and unfolds at different historical paces (Rose, 2006). As I have tried to argue and demonstrate throughout the course of this paper, Rabinow's essay proposes that we should not begin our investigations with preconceived notions of what patients' organisations, biotechnology firms, lay persons or scientists are, but rather to focus on the series of practices and forms through which they are assembled at different sites and on various scales of analysis. It could be said that the institutions, assemblages, and practices that make up contemporary social formations are made and transformed through present day activities. However, practices, can take on enduring forms: these forms are assembled out of a combination of old and new practices. As a heuristic device, Rabinow was concerned with exploring the bonds between labour and life, life and language,

language and labour to see where they would lead. One place where this has led me, is to consider Myozyme as an examplar of biosociality.

In considering Myozyme as an exemplar of biosociality, I want to move away from the almost exclusive sociological and anthropological consideration of this term to refer to the forms of activism characteristic of contemporary genetic advocacy groups. Myozyme, as a treatment created through the genetic modification of CHO cells so that they are capable of excreting human acid-alpha-glucocidase that can be successfully used to alter the natural biology of Pompe disease so that it is in accordance with cultural conceptions of health and lifespan is emblematic of biosociality. This therapy further represents an instance where we can see the refraction of the practices of life, labour and language on a number of sites and at a variety of scales of analysis. Myozyme is a combination of science, ethics, marketing, capital, nature, culture, legislation, intellectual property and a brand.

Thinking about Myozyme as a brand makes it possible to consider how the fields of life, labour, and language may be undergoing a transition from being characterised by finitude to what Gilles Deleuze terms the 'unlimited-finite'. Political economy provides a useful starting point for such an analysis. Conventional economics considered the production process as involving the development of a product, its introduction to markets, and its subsequent branding to help distinguish it from other products on the market. In the case of Myozyme, this temporal sequence was disrupted – the product was branded even before it was available on the market in Europe and the United States. Furthermore, the branding of this therapy is not about distinguishing it from other products on the market – Myozyme is the only product on the market. The link between a product and brand is further ruptured when we begin to consider that branding can be used to help distinguish firms such as Genzyme. So what is a brand? A series of practices. Of course, branding is not new, it has a long historical lineage, especially in the pharmaceutical industry. However, branding is being adapted to suit contemporary purposes. Branding practices are no longer intimately tied to a product, but to establishing a series of relationships over time with entities such as firms, universities, philanthropic organisations, customers, stakeholders, physicians, the public and so on (Lury, 2004).

Myozyme as a brand refracts and pleats the fields of life, labour and language onto one another. Myozyme is a treatment for a severe disease and a potential platform for producing more efficacious therapies for LSD through Genzyme's acquisition of Novazyme's proprietary technologies. It is also a product of and an entity which participates in giving form to markets in unmet medical needs. Myozyme will contribute to the generation of value for Genzyme through the global sales of this therapy, by improving the health and quality of life of persons affected by Pompe disease, and by contributing to this firm's image as an organisation which can fulfil the medical needs of persons whose diseases have been orphaned by medicine and the market. The realisation of the economic, somatic, and social value contained in Myozyme requires the mobilisation of a range of signs, symbols, and practices. It requires patients and physicians who understand the disease and its treatment modalities, the processes through which Myozyme is manufactured, the clinical trial procedures through which the efficacy and safety of this therapy were established, and the creation of a website for the Pompe community (see www.pompe.com for details of all of the aforementioned). As a brand, Myozyme requires the establishment and formation of a diverse series of relationships over time: these relationships include the expectations Genzyme mobilised around the development of a therapy for Pompe disease over the past several years; the successful recruitment and participation of infants, children and adults in the clinical trials Genzyme conducted to enable this therapy to be approved for marketing authorisation in Europe and the United States; the creation of a range of patient/customer education and support tools to assist persons who will receive this therapy; to the creation of expectations that Genzyme will develop even better therapies for persons affected by Pompe disease in the years to come. Myozyme provides ample opportunity to reflect on how nature and culture, time and space are folded and collapsed upon themselves in contemporary social formations.

In thinking through the implications of Myozyme as an entity which is neither opaque or has a perfected form – or what Deleuze has termed the unlimited-finite – I believe that it is important to begin reconsidering how sociology produces accounts of science and technology. Throughout the course of this paper, I have tried to show how Genzyme generates economic value through a diverse range of practices, rather than from solely intervening upon vital life processes. I have been concerned with the processes of capitalisation that have brought Myozyme into being and how it contributes to the generation of a range of economic, somatic and social values that in many ways extend beyond the purview of Genzyme's corporate practices. In thinking about how Myozyme generates economic value, it is important to query conventional explanations of drug development in terms of a movement from the laboratory to the clinic. Alternatively, we need to look at the multiple pathways, sites and practices through which therapies emerge and generate value. This makes it possible to think about how the creation of Myozyme owes as much to science as to the range of practices and practitioners who helped to bring this brand into being – from marketing professionals to the patients who participated in clinical trials. Sociologists need to develop new discursive practices and to retool their economic concepts so that they are suitable for thinking about and accounting for the contributions of diverse scientific practitioners and technological innovators. Perhaps we need a new conception of what science is and the persons who are authorised to practise it.

Acknowledgements

I would like to thank Ayo Walhberg, Chris Hamilton, Linsey McGoey, Scott Vrecko, Shirlene Badger, Paul Rabinow and Javier Lezaun for their very helpful comments on earlier versions of this paper. I would also especially like to thank Cecilia D'Felice who taught me a thing or two about affect and care of the self. This research was conducted through the support provided by a Wellcome Trust Postdoctoral Research Fellowship.

Notes

1 While doctors had initially diagnosed the Crowleys' children with the infantile form of Pompe disease where children usually die within the first year of life, they have an extremely rare form of the disease, where the life expectancy extends to adolescence.

2 'We're battling against nature and time', said Crowley … 'But to cure any disease, no matter how rare and simple, takes money, because money buys science'. In terms of Children Pompe Foundation 'We want to find the most effective cure as quickly as possible for our children and about 1,000 other children in the United States with all forms of Pompe disease', Crowley said (D'Aurizio, 1999a). 'It is as much a race against time as it is against nature', Crowley said. 'I have no doubt we'll beat nature. I have talked to enough scientists around the world to know this disease will be cured and cured very quickly' (D'Aurizio, 1999b).

3 'Crowley said that $6 billion is computed by taking the 50 lysosomal storage diseases and multiplying that number by the number of patients and the average price per therapy, which will be approximately $100,000 per patient, per year' (Carter, 2000).

4 'I've always said all along that my personal interests and the interests of Novazyme and the interests of any parent of any patient are perfectly aligned, and that's to bring the most effective therapy to as many patients as quickly as possible', Crowley said. 'So for my children, Megan and Patrick, and for thousands of children like them around the world, we think our drug will provide fundamental enhancement to their quality of life with the hope that it could potentially completely reverse the disease, which would be a dream for a lot of people' (Carter, 2000).

5 A problem that confronted the production of Ceredase was that it required using up to 22,000 human placentas to produce sufficient enzyme to treat a single patient for a year. The production of Ceredase was not only limited by the supply of human placentas, but it also created the potential for infection through contaminated placentas (Office of Technology Assessment, 1992).

6 This medico-industrial environment must not only satisfy the demands of the cells which live in them, but must also comply with a range of regulations that is encompassed by the term Good Manufacturing Practice guidelines.

References

Anand, G. (2003) 'For his sick kids, a father struggles to develop a cure', *Wall Street Journal*, New York.

Anand, G. (2006) *The Cure: How a Father Raised $100 Million – and Bucked the Medical Establishment – in a Quest to Save His Children*, New York: HarperCollins.

Ashton, G. (2001) 'Growing pains for biopharmaceuticals', *Nature Biotechnology*, 19, 4: 307–11.

Beard, R.L. (2004) 'Advocating voice: organisational, historical and social milieux of the Alzheimer's disease movement', *Sociology of Health and Illness*, 26, 6: 797–819.

Brown, N. (2003) 'Hope against hype – accountability in biopasts, presents and futures', *Science Studies*, 16, 2: 3–21.

Brown, N., Rappert, B. and Webster, A. (2000) *Contested Futures: A Sociology of Prospective Techno-Science*, Aldershot: Ashgate.

Carter, R. (2000) 'Seeking the Holy Grail of chronic therapies', *The Journal Record*, Oklahoma.

Couzin, J. (2005) 'Advocating, the clinical way', *Science*, 13 May: 940–2.

D'Aurizio, E. (1999a) 'Little lives in the balance: parents work to find cure for two tots rare disease', *The Record*, Bergen County, NJ.

D'Aurizio, E. (1999b) 'A spark of hope in fight for their lives: father of sick children presses for cure', *The Record*, Bergen County, NJ.

Deleuze, G. (1988) *Foucault*, Minneapolis, MN: University of Minnesota Press.

Deleuze, G. (1995) 'Postscript on control societies', in Deleuze, G. (ed.) *Negotiations: 1972–1990*, New York: Columbia University Press.

Exceptional Parent (2000a) 'Strength in the face of adversity, part 1', *The Exceptional Parent*, 1 February.

Exceptional Parent (2000b) 'Strength in the face of adversity, part 2', *The Exceptional Parent*, 1 March.

Haffner, M.E. (2003) 'The current environment in orphan drug development', *Drug Information Journal*, 37: 373–9.

Haffner, M.E., Whitley, J. and Moses, M. (2002) 'Two decades of orphan drug development', *Nature Reviews Drug Discovery*, 1, 10: 821–5.

Heath, D. (1998) 'Locating genetic knowledge: picturing Marfan Syndrome and its travelling constituencies', *Science, Technology, and Human Values*, 23, 1: 71–97.

Hedgecoe, A. and Martin, P. (2003) 'The drugs don't work: expectations and the shaping of pharmacogenetics', *Social Studies of Science*, 33, 3: 327–64.

Henderson, L. and Kitzinger, J. (1999) 'The human drama of genetics: "hard" and "soft" media representations of inherited breast cancer', *Sociology of Health and Illness*, 21, 5: 560–78.

Hughes, H.M. (1968) *News and the Human Interest Story*, New York: Greenwood Press.

Latour, B. (1987) *Science in Action: How to Follow Scientists and Engineers through Society*, Cambridge, MA: Harvard University Press.

Lury, C. (2004) *Brands: The Logos of the Global Economy*, London: Routledge.

Novas, C. (2006) 'The political economy of hope: patients' organizations, science and biovalue', *BioSocieties*, 1, 3: 289–305.

Office of Technology Assessment (1992) 'Federal and private roles in the development and provision of alglucerase therapy for Gaucher disease'.

Petersen, A. (2001) 'Biofantasies: genetics and medicine in the print news media', *Social Science and Medicine*, 52, 8: 1255–68.

PR Newswire (2000) 'Novazyme Pharmaceuticals announces multiple research programs for treatment of lysosomal storage disorders;' *PR Newswire*, 6 June.

PR Newswire (2003) 'SBI and company develops website for Genzyme to raise awareness of Pompe disease', *PR Newswire*, 21 May.

Rabinow, P. (1996) 'Artificiality and enlightenment: from sociobiology to biosociality', *Essays on the Anthropology of Reason*, Princeton NJ: Princeton University Press.

Rapp, R. (2000) 'Extra chromosomes and blue tulips: medico-familial interpretations', in Lock, M., Young, A. and Cambrosio, A. (eds) *Living and Working with the New Medical Technologies: Intersections of Inquiry*, Cambridge: Cambridge University Press.

Rapp, R. (2003) 'Cell life and death, child life and death: genomic horizons, genetic diseases, family stories', in Franklin, S. and Lock, M.M. (eds) *Remaking Life and Death: Toward an Anthropology of the Biosciences*, Oxford: James Currey.

Robbins-Roth, C. (2000) *From Alchemy to IPO: the Business of Biotechnology*, Cambridge, MA: Perseus.

Rose, N. (2006) *The Politics of Life Itself: Biomedicine, Power, and Subjectivity in the Twenty-First Century*, Princeton, NJ: Princeton University Press.

Rose, N. and Novas, C. (2005) 'Biological citizenship', in Ong, A. and Collier, S. (eds) *Global Assemblages: Technology, Politics, and Ethics as Anthropological Problems*, Malden, MA: Blackwell.

Salter, M.S. and Green, D.B. (2001) 'Tracking stocks at Genzyme', *Harvard Business School Case Study*.

Savage, M. (2005) 'The popularity of bureaucracy: involvement in voluntary organisations', in Du Gay, P. (ed.) *The Values of Bureaucracy*, Oxford: Oxford University Press.

Shostak, S. (2004) 'Environmental justice and genomics: acting on the futures of environmental health', *Science as Culture*, 13, 4: 539–61.

Stockdale, A. (1999) 'Waiting for the cure: mapping the social relations of human gene therapy research', *Sociology of Health and Illness*, 21, 5: 579–96.

Stockdale, A. and Terry, S.F. (2002) 'Advocacy groups and the new genetics', in Alper, J.S., Ard, C., Asch, A., Beckwith, J., Conrad, P. and Geller, L.N. (eds) *The Double-Edged Helix: Social Implications of Genetics in a Diverse Society*, Baltimore, MD: Johns Hopkins University Press.

Terry, S.F. (2003) 'Learning Genetics', *Health Affairs*, 22, 5: 166–70.

Waldby, C. (2000) *The Visible Human Project: Informatic Bodies and Posthuman Medicine*, London and New York: Routledge.

Waldby, C. (2002) 'Stem cells, tissue cultures and the production of biovalue', *Health: An Interdisciplinary Journal for the Social Study of Health, Illness and Medicine*, 6, 3: 305–23.

Watson, N. (2003) 'This Dutchman is flying: maverick biotech firm Genzyme is winning big profits from a contrarian strategy', *Fortune*, 23 June.

8   Biocapital as an emergent form of life

Speculations on the figure of the experimental subject

Kaushik Sunder Rajan

I

The value of Paul Rabinow's concept of biosociality, I believe, lies in the way in which it functions, at the same time, with an absolute specificity and with a productive indeterminacy. This indeterminacy has already been pointed to by the editors. One of the rationales for this volume, they suggest, is that biosociality is a term that is generative of so many different directions of empirical inquiry. It is a concept that serves less as a definition than as a provocation. It signifies a problem space that is opened up for the human sciences by the biological sciences, where emergences in the latter place a whole range of philosophical, conceptual and methodological questions – concerning, for instance, questions of the social, of culture, of political economy, of ethics and of governance – at stake. And it is a provocation that has, for the most part, been taken up in particular ways – as indicated in this volume, oftentimes by looking at the ways in which social identity gets reconfigured through new biomedical technologies.

But it is the specificity of the concept that interests me equally, and relates to the conjunctures in relation to which the notion of biosociality was born, and the quite different conjunctures in relation to which it can be applied. Biosociality is an incredibly generative concept, but it is one that needs to be situated historically and in terms of modes of production and what Michael Fischer (drawing on Raymond Williams, Ludwig Wittgenstein and Emmanuel Levinas) calls "forms of life" (Fischer 2003). I wish to situate it thus in this essay, using ethnographic material from Bombay, and Williams' heuristic of residual, dominant and emergent formations as a means to locate the case that I narrate (Williams 1973).

This case is of experimental subject formation in Parel, one of the mill districts of Bombay. This is a story that I have already narrated in greater detail elsewhere, so will only summarize in schematic form here.[1] Briefly – I am concerned here with the setting up of a clinical research organization (CRO) called Wellquest in Parel. Wellquest is part of an institutional triad that consisted, in addition to the CRO, of a hospital (Wellspring) and a genome company (Genomed). All three entities were seeded by an Indian pharmaceutical company, Nicholas Piramal India Limited (NPIL). Joint equity in Genomed was held by the Indian state through one of its public laboratories, the Center for Biochemical Technology

(CBT, subsequently renamed the Institute for Genomics and Integrative Biology, IGIB).[2] These entities were formed in 2000, but Genomed has recently shut down. Wellspring and Wellquest, however, are still in existence, making the latter one of the older and more established CROs in India today.

Wellquest and Genomed interested me as part of my earlier project on post-genomics in the US and India, because they presented a melding together of new forms of biomedical and corporate enterprise that was surrounding both the sequencing of the human genome in the US, and India's serious attempt to enter into the global genomics marketplace (which involved a larger embrace of what Indian state and corporate actors would call a "culture of innovation"). The particular locus of biomedical collaboration between Wellquest and Genomed was around pharmacogenomics, which involves testing to correlate drug response of individuals to their genetics. Pharmacogenomics is the biomedical activity that most directly sees a coming together of genomic epistemologies and technologies with biomedical and market considerations in drug development. It is a potentially valuable tool for biotechnology and pharmaceutical companies, as it would allow the stratification of patient populations in terms of drug response.[3] The contracting clients that Wellquest and Genomed were looking for quite explicitly included Western biotech and pharmaceutical companies.[4] Regardless of the local ecologies within which certain enterprises were emerging, or their subsequent success or failure in market terms, these emergent assemblages were of empirical and conceptual interest.

But the local ecologies made them far more interesting, and turned out to be essential to elucidate in order to generate any sort of thick contextualization of the sorts of emergences that I was seeing. And this concerned the fact that Wellspring was located in Parel. The textile mills, which formed the basis of Bombay's emergence as a center of capital in India, have been slowly eviscerated over the last thirty years, with a number of mills shutting down.[5] Most of the unemployed workers currently work as security guards in new shopping malls, or as street hawkers. They also, according to scientists I have talked to at Wellspring, are the subjects most commonly recruited into clinical trials at Wellquest.

The potentially biosocial situation here, quite obviously, concerns the emergence of biomedical capabilities in India and the recruitment of experimental subjects into clinical trials. Given that this situation emerges in the context of a market venture, it also concerns biocapital. But the location of this situation, which provides it with its specificity, speaks to two other circuits of capital. The textile industry is a form of manufacturing capitalism; the evisceration of this industry is because of a larger structural transformation underway in Bombay (and in India more generally) towards investments in both the global service industry and in local real estate, both of which are forms of speculative capitalism. In Williams' terms, I argue that industrial-scale textile manufacturing, speculative real estate and clinical trials constitute, respectively, the residual, dominant and emergent formations in Bombay today.

Each of these structural formations, from the perspective of both the workers and of capital, has associated socialities of action, and it is these which I wish to trace and interrogate. What are the shared social identifications that one sees in Bombay in this intertwining of three structural forms of capitalism? And what might we understand, about both biosociality and the social formations of capital, through an unpacking of these social identifications?

Using the case of Parel as a springboard, I wish to ask the question of the sorts of identity formation that take shape amongst these mill workers-turned-experimental subjects. Further, I wish to suggest that the displacements and reconfigurations that new emergences in biomedical research bring about here occur not just through technical and epistemic emergences, but crucially along with emergences in new forms, locales and strategies of capital accumulation, and have constitutive to them a structural violence. I locate this structural violence in the necessary constitution of experimental subjects for clinical research that attends these technologies.

II

Before moving on to the empirical substance of this paper, I wish to spend some time considering sociality as an analytic concept. I make two arguments here. The first is that sociality cannot be taken for granted – it never always already exists, but has to be brought into being. The *formation* of sociality can be registered and studied either historically (which was Karl Marx's method in reading political economy in the context of social relations of production) or through an epochal analysis (Michel Foucault's "archaeological" method, employed especially in his earlier works). More importantly, sociality can also not be assumed structurally or antagonistically. In other words, even if social relations of production apparently pit "classes" of people in a potentially antagonistic relationship to one another, such antagonism only manifests in historically specific ways.

The second is that sociality always already implies subjectivity. Subjectivity becomes the crucial analytic through which sociality (which sometimes forms, and sometimes does not) can be studied. "The biosocial subject" is one whose subjectivity is transformed into a sociality, and this transformation constitutes a crucial *political* moment. It is the point at which subjectivity as *subjection* becomes potentially or actually transformed into subjectivity as sociopolitical *agency*.[6] If one is to ask the question of biosociality in the context of Parel, it is essential to first elucidate the sorts of subject-formation that are taking place there in the articulations of industrial, speculative and bio-capital. From the perspective of mill workers-turned-experimental subjects, identity formation is apparently not biosocial at all, but rather constituted (in various historically implicated ways) along lines of class, locality and nationalism. I wish to situate this case of class-based identity formation against that of a risk-based identity formation that forms the contours of biosociality.

Foucault's exposition of biopolitics is a diagnosis of the ways in which life becomes the explicit center of political calculation in a modernist rationality (Foucault 1990 [1978]). The mode of biopolitical governance has increasingly been through an articulation of risk. Risk is a crucial heuristic for Rabinow in his essay on biosociality. Reading Robert Castel, he traces the way in which a discourse of risk becomes central both to the biosciences and to modernist configurations of the social, leading to individual self-fashioning ("the promotion of working on oneself in a continuous fashion"),[7] further leading to an "efficient and adaptable subject.[8]

I wish in this essay to push this notion of risk, by placing it in different analytic registers. For Castel, whose analysis derives from a study of psychiatric epistemology, risk operates in relation to technologies of self-fashioning.[9] In the process, risk is not merely individuating, but also provides the epistemic conditions of possibility for certain kinds of shared social identification to emerge. This is a crucial analytic for biosociality as a notion to base itself on, and indeed mirrors the ways in which Ulrich Beck argues for the formation of new sociopolitical alliances based on the knowledge of environmental risk, as a marker of 1980s European "risk society" (Beck 1986).

As Francois Ewald has shown, however, risk operates not just as an epistemology of self-fashioning, but also quite directly as a form of capital (Ewald 1991). One sees this most typically in the insurance industry, the subject of Ewald's analysis, as an industry whose calculus of market value involves calculating life itself. But it is central to the dynamics of speculative capital writ large, to the point where, certainly in the United States, the calculation of market risk (and in relation to that, the potential for market growth) is far more crucial to corporate valuation than the calculation of revenues or profits. Therefore, if risk operates as an epistemology of self-fashioning, then it also operates as an epistemology of market valuation. This becomes particularly interesting in the case of the pharmaceutical and biotechnology industries, intensified through new emergences in the life sciences such as genomics that specifically diagnose risk profiles, since both calculations of risk are at stake – on the one hand, of the patient-in-waiting's risk of future disease (providing future market potential for companies in the business of therapeutic development), and on the other, of the corporation's market risk (based in failures in drug development or the recall of drugs after marketing because of adverse events; risks to market share because of competitors, especially acute when drugs come off patent leading to the possibility of generic competition; or constant risks of public relations disasters and state legislation, especially around questions of drug pricing).[10]

There is a third register at which I wish to analyze risk in this essay, and that is *as labor*. Rabinow's analytic attempt in his biosociality essay is to push the ways in which the interaction of life and labor changes through new emergences in the life sciences. Reconfigurations in understandings of life itself are implicated in new forms of labor – one that leads to new forms of sociality, but equally one that is individuated and not based on a structurally given social formation such as class. A major form that such "laboring" takes in the context of biosociality – anticipated by Rabinow, and fleshed out in rich empirical detail in a number of essays in this volume – is that of patient advocacy. But I am interested in another type of constitutive labor that is part of the assemblage of biotechnical knowledge production, and that is the labor performed by the experimental subject – a subject-position that is based neither in "working on oneself in a continuous fashion," nor is "efficient and adaptable," but is rather *merely risked*. I wish to locate this "merely risked" subject-position not outside the circuits of biosociality, but rather as a constitutive condition of possibility for the efficient and adaptable biosocial subject to exist.

Before speaking specifically of experimental subjects in Parel (or in India more generally), it is important to understand the place of clinical experimentation in contemporary biomedicine writ large. This involves understanding both biomedical and market rationalities. The biomedical rationality concerns the specific ways in which humans respond to drugs, something which can never be extrapolated well enough from laboratory and animal experiments without conducting separate, independent experiments on humans to test for drug safety and efficacy. In other words, *to the extent that therapeutic development constitutes a desired end-point of biomedical practice*, clinical research is constitutive to the experimental form of the life sciences. The market impacts this in significant ways, because clinical trials also constitute the most expensive part of the drug development process, a process that according to industry estimates costs nearly a billion dollars per new therapeutic molecule (di Masi *et al.* 1991).[11] Any way in which clinical trials costs can be reduced, therefore, is seen as crucial to reduce the overall costs of drug development, which leads to the potential attraction of Third World sites as outsourcing destinations for such research. Therefore, there is a productive logic, tying into both biomedical and market factors, that necessitates clinical research, and that sees a cost advantage to taking that research to the Third World. There are a couple of crucial issues to unpack here before I move on to situate this productive logic in the specific context of clinical research capacity-building in India.

The first – to the extent that therapeutic development constitutes a desired end-point of biomedical practice, to what extent does it do so? At one level, this is a question that demands historical and empirical specificity, and one of the crucial moments of Rabinow's essay on biosociality is his identification of the way in which, in the case of genomics, *diagnostic* potential supersedes *therapeutic* potential. It is far easier for gene sequences to act as markers for disease than it is to use those markers to design a therapeutic molecule, let alone manufacture a functional therapeutic molecule that can act at a genetic or protein level to modulate a disease. And therefore, if one is to understand the epistemic reconfigurations that genomics brings about, it is crucial to look towards diagnostics rather than therapeutics as an immediate "end-point," both in terms of biomedical intervention and as a potentially reliable business model.[12] Therefore, to the extent that genomics reconfigures biomedical practice (something that could only be speculated upon at the time of the biosociality essay), it is arguably not therapy that is the name of the game at all. Indeed, the "form" of therapy that is envisioned through genomics, personalized medicine, is not conceived of in terms of therapeutic molecules as much as it is in terms of an ensemble of diagnostic and prophylactic practices (some of them necessarily involving therapeutic consumption) that has prevention of disease as its core rationality.

At another level, however, therapeutic potential overdetermines biomedical rationality. And so, if one considers the monetary investments that go into biomedical research, whether public or private, they are invariably animated by a promise and/or hope of eventual therapeutic development. So too, indeed, are the affective investments, on the part of patient advocacy groups, for instance. If at an epistemic register, genomics opens up diagnostic potential most directly, then at a subjective register – the way in which genomics is invested in, valuated and consumed – therapy remains very much the name of the game. And that means that the constitutive importance of clinical research as a crucial node in the biomedical chain remains.

The second issue to think about in terms of the productive logic of biomedicine and its relationship to clinical research on the one hand, and biosociality on the other, concerns *scale*. Rabinow's conception of life science research in his biosociality essay is almost entirely situated within the *laboratory*; translating those laboratory results into the *clinic* is a crucial scaling endeavor. As Anna Tsing has argued, the scaling of practice (not just experimental practice) is never seamless, but always frictioned (Tsing 2004). The scaling of laboratory research to the clinic is similarly frictioned. This is in part because certain experimental variables cannot be adequately accounted for before the act of scaling itself. Most evident amongst these incalculable variables is human response to drugs – as mentioned earlier, no amount of *in vitro* or animal studies can adequately predict the way a drug will respond in a human subject. Animal tests, therefore, at best form a sort of experimental triage – if a drug is found to be excessively toxic to rats, for instance, it is unlikely to be tested at all on humans. The earliest stages of human clinical trials are one of the few moments in biomedical experimentation when a hypothesis-driven research paradigm completely breaks down – one *has* to see what the drug does to a trial subject before one can draw any further conclusions about its likely safety or efficacy, or what an ideal dose might be.

In addition to the general unpredictability of human response to drugs is the specific unpredictability of response of particular individuals or populations. There are genetic variations in individuals' response to drugs (that largely have to do with the differential rates of drug metabolism by different individuals, and which in turn largely depends on the activity of the Cytochrome P-450 group of drug metabolizing enzymes). And there are environmental factors that will cause differential drug response between individuals and populations, such as different diets, or the number of drugs that one is already taking.

One level at which scaling from laboratory to clinic becomes frictioned, then, is in terms of the variability to be found between human and animal response to drugs, and in drug response between different human individuals and populations. But another level of friction is added if part of the scale-making involves taking a trial global. What a globalization of a clinical trial involves is an extreme level of coordination and standardization. This has to occur at the level of data management, medical history taking and record keeping, the actual trial protocol, and also regulatory practice.

The experimental subject of clinical research in a global clinical trial, therefore, is formed consequent to market rationalities that press biomedical research towards therapeutic development; cost rationalities that seek to reduce the expense of clinical trials; biomedical rationalities that encourage the inclusion of a wide range of population groups in many forms of clinical research (though this would depend on the specificities of particular research projects); the inherent experimental uncertainty of translating laboratory research up to humans (and the risk to experimental subjects that attends this uncertainty); and the imperatives of standardization – of clinical practice, of experimental protocol implementation, of data management, and of regulatory guidelines.[13] In addition, as I show below, such a subject is formed consequent to strategic and tactical state and business rationalities and to larger structural transformations in political economic systems. This is the assemblage that I wish to unpack in greater detail in the substance of this paper, asking all the while how biosociality might take shape within such a constellation of systemic forces and historical and global conjunctures.

III

My earlier accounts of the experimental subjectivity of the mill workers of Parel as a consequence of changing structures of capitalism (away from manufacturing, towards speculative) were oriented primarily from the perspective of capital (Sunder Rajan 2005, 2006). In this essay, I wish to investigate this experimental subjectivity, and the forms of social identification that emerge or endure amongst the mill workers of Parel, from the perspective of labor. For this, I turn to conversations I have had with mill workers' unions. The mill districts of Bombay are amongst the most highly unionized parts of India, and indeed formed the fulcrum of the rise of the trade union movement in India in the early part of the twentieth century.

I wish here to elaborate upon a conversation with Datta Isswalkar, who leads the Girni Kamgar Sangarsh Samiti (GKSS, literally meaning workers' struggle union) in order to emphasize questions of subjectivity and sociality as they emerge (or do not) in the context of residual, dominant and emergent formations of capitalism. GKSS is one of the two major unions in the mill districts, and the one that is more oppositional to the developments happening in the districts. The locus of this opposition, as elaborated upon in the transcripts below, concerns the consequences of real estate development in the mill lands, and the payment of back-wages to workers.[14] Earlier struggles focused on reopening closed mills, but that is now largely seen as a lost cause. The crucial issue now is whether the mills can be torn down to make way for high rise apartments and shopping malls, given that the mill districts are located in the heart of Bombay (geographically analogous to where Grand Central Station might be located in respect to Manhattan), and therefore represents prime real estate. The reason why this is so important to the workers is because of the question of tenancy rights. As part of the development of the textile mills in the 1920s and 1930s, the then-British mill owners built a series of one-floor tenements called *chawls*, which housed the mill workers. The *chawls* do not just provide the workers with shelter, but also became an integral part of the social fabric of the mill districts. The built environment of the mill districts provided the conditions of possibility for certain sorts of organizing, both around labor (the trade union movement), and also nationalist organizing as part of the freedom struggle in the 1930s and 1940s. In other words, the urban environment of the mill districts had everything to do with the formation of *working class consciousness* – this was never an essentialist consequence of a structural subject-position within work (and, as I will argue subsequently, never has been throughout industrial capitalism), but was rather itself consequent to particular "regimes of living" (Collier and Lakoff 2005). The unions, along with allied urban and environmental NGOs, were able to get a legal stay on real estate development in the mill districts through a Bombay High Court order, but that was overturned in March 2006 by the Indian Supreme Court, thereby paving the way for the mills (and the *chawls*) to be torn down for real estate development.

It is in this context that I wish to elaborate upon my conversation with Isswalkar. I am interested here in working through a problem-space as it unfolds through the lens of what is, in this case, a social consciousness that is resolutely working class, and that is structurally tied in to a particular locality in historically very specific ways.[15]

Excerpts of interview transcript with Datta Isswalkar, Girni Kamgar Sangarsh Samiti, 30 July 2004

Isswalkar starts his account by elaborating upon the historical and structural transformations that have been underway in Bombay:

> Whatever development (of Bombay) happened was through the cotton industry, the first industries that were made here were the textile mills. The industry of this city started from there. Workers came from all over the country ... Now what is happening is that these people want to change this city from an industrial city to a, what do you say, they want to make it into a business centre. They want to make it a centre of commerce.

These structural transformations, predictably, have had adverse consequences for the mill workers, whose interests have not been adequately taken into account:

> The question that arises is for these people who have come from all these places, what will get made for them? You want to make this like Hong Kong or Singapore, in this service center, in this centre of commerce, will space be made (for these people), this is our question for the government. We have no opposition to this. You want to make it into Hong Kong, make it like New York. But this working class that has come here, are you making space for it? Why not? In this day what we see is 600 acres of mill land. On this land 250,000 workers are working, two and a half lakhs. So if you are going to use

this land for housing, where will these people go? It may be that then these people will end up working as hawkers, but they are not even being allowed to sit as hawkers, because it is said that this makes the streets noisy, that it makes it hard to create parking spaces. So what I am saying is, this urban transformation that they want to make, this development that they want to do, this development is not in the benefit of these workers, it is going to take them on the road to ruin. This is what we have to say today.[16]

These consequences have resulted in enormous strain on and alienation of workers, leading either to their joining gangs and becoming a part of the notorious Bombay underworld, or in the case of older workers, quite often committing suicide:

Many, many workers have committed suicide. As I have told you, in Khatau Mills, how many people have killed themselves? Because their salaries were stopped, they did not get their dues, what will they do? And who does commit suicide? The ones who are over 40 years of age, the ones who have children, who cannot bear to see the state of their children. That is why they commit suicide. The youth doesn't commit suicide. They will become gangsters, won't they? They will take things. They will steal. But the people who have families, who cannot bear to see, they can't bear to see you see, they can't feed their children. Therefore they commit suicide. This is why no young farmers die, just take a look. The youth turn into gangsters, don't they? They won't commit suicide, they will steal. They will become gangsters. So this is what is happening, because of globalization, for farmers and workers this has become too much. All these suicides that you are seeing in front of you, all of this has to be thought about, if the city to go in a different direction, then you should see what all happens because of that.[17]

The only way in which this alienation can be prevented is through the organization of the workers, and this leads to the setting of agendas and strategies for union activities:

One thing that has happened is in the textile mills, the textile mills have been closing down. So it came to our attention that for the workers, for the youth, there is now the challenge of unemployment. So we got scared, where will the youth go now? The first place he will go is to the gangsters. So we thought we should make an organization, of unemployed youth, and present to the government the fact that we don't want to become gangsters, give us work. If you want to make the city commercial, you want to make it for business, then I too should have the wherewithal to do business, shouldn't I? If the youth of this place want to do their own business, something small, if he wants to run a small shop, then why don't you make the arrangements for that? For example, we say give him a shop at low cost, then he too will do business won't he? ...

As part of this workers' struggle, we have made one demand of the government, that on this mill land, for instance this hospital is coming up, so there will be jobs created within it, ward boys, nurses, watchmen, people in different labs to conduct various tests, this is all work that can be done by the children of mill workers. So the government has passed a law, which says that whatever employment opportunities get created on mill land, work has to be given to family members of mill workers. This job the government has done ... Now we have to follow up on it. What will happen is that we will register mill workers, but how will mill owners know that they have to give work to mill workers, that this is the law? That will just remain on the books, won't it? So we have to tell the owners, and tell the mill workers' youth, their family members, that the government has made this law for you. That is the work that we have to do.

According to Isswalkar, the evisceration of the textile industry itself was not purely due to structural transformations in capitalism that led to the gradual decline of the mills, but rather has been due to the actions of the mill owners, who have themselves tried to run their own mills into the ground. The reason for this:

As I told you at the beginning, the atmosphere of the city, the development of the city, if it has to be turned into a business center, then industry has to go, doesn't it? So first everything about this city was industrial, there were chemical industries, there were textile industries. And the other thing is that in this country, in India, the land value in Bombay city is the highest. So the owners thought, since the mill owners are landlords as well, they own lots of land. You need a lot of land for the textile industry. They own about 600 acres of land. So what did they think? That this industry I can run anywhere else. If I can earn millions of rupees per day on this land, then their character is such, they are only going to think of the business they can accrue from this. That I can get so much money from this land, which I couldn't get even if I ran the textile industry for a hundred years. So they are engaged in dealing in the land itself. This is the question of mills in Bombay is the question of the mill lands. If you take the lands away, then these millionaires have nothing left. You ask any millionaire, Mafatlal or anyone else, that if the government took this land from you what would you have left, they would have nothing left. So the mill lands have become for them, have become a type of capital. And basically these people are selling it, making money from it. This is how it is.

There are a few things that I wish to emphasize from these transcripts for the purposes of this essay. The first concerns the structural diagnosis of transformation in modes and relations of production, a larger historical transformation from industrial to speculative capitalism in Bombay, one locus of which becomes the mill lands, thereby implicating mill workers. This is seen, as Isswalkar emphasized early in the conversation, as a *working class* issue. The issues at stake here are labor and, given the crucial place of land in this struggle, tenancy.

The second concerns the symptomatic *absence* of any knowledge of the experiments occurring on mill workers. This in spite of the fact that Isswalkar is aware of the existence of Wellspring hospital, which he refers to during the conversation as one possible place where unemployed workers could perhaps be given employment, as watchmen or ward boys or lab technicians. Indeed, every time I mentioned the issue of mill workers as experimental subjects to members of workers unions, or other people involved in demanding rights for the mill workers, I encountered a lack of knowledge about this situation. The only people who seemed to know that mill workers were getting recruited into the trials were scientists at Wellquest. This in itself is not surprising – the identities of trial volunteers are never made public, and I have found it impossible to talk to trial subjects themselves through the aegis of clinical research organizations.[18] What is interesting for me here is that shared biological identification (in terms of experimental subjectivity) is *not* the locus of sociality, even though people getting recruited into trials seem to be coming from similar class backgrounds, and from a fairly circumscribed locality.

On the face of it, this conversation can be read as having nothing to do with biosociality. It could be read as a different problem, relating to a different circuit of capital, one that has to do with the intersection of industrial manufacturing with speculative real estate. But I wish to argue that the insertion of Wellspring into this ecology makes this story entirely about biosociality; or at least forces us to trace how the insertion of biocapital into a situation of industrial and speculative capital impacts both the logics of industrial and speculative capital, and forces us to consider biosociality and biocapital in terms of the structural conjunctures within which they emerge.

IV

So far in this essay, I have attempted to juxtapose logics of clinical trials within biomedical political economy and epistemology against shifting logics and processes of global capital as it touches down in Bombay. In the process, my attempt is to show that biocapital is one key index of "capitalism" in all its multiple manifestations. Some empirical situations (pertaining, for instance, to genomics, drug development or clinical trials) could unequivocally be "about" biocapital, while others could be about other forms of capital, for instance industrial manufacturing or real estate speculation. Biocapital, therefore, is a specific institutional form of capitalism, driven by particular epistemic rationalities and strategic and tactical actions. But it is simultaneously indexical of "capitalism" as a larger structural construct because it contains within it logics of other forms of capital (drug development, for instance, depends both on industrial-scale manufacturing and on huge amounts of financial speculation), and because it articulates with other forms of capital in particular places and times in contingent yet historically shaped ways.

Similarly, I see Rabinow's biosociality as one key index of biocapital. But his accent on the efficient, adaptable, self-fashioning biosocial subject actually only indexes part of the situation – that having to do with those subjects who are configured or act as *consumers* – while naturalizing the experimental subjects. In this section, I wish to elaborate upon this argument by considering the socialities implicated in the residual, dominant and emergent structural formations of industrial, speculative and bio-capital in Bombay today. My argument is that these socialities are not symmetrical from the perspective of workers and of capital, and this asymmetry has to be taken into account if one is to understand experimental subjectivity in the context of biosociality.

The residual sociality from the perspective of workers, pertaining to histories of industrial capitalism, is seen in the endurance of the trade union movement in Bombay. The textile unions in Bombay are amongst the oldest in India and have been active since the early part of the twentieth century, involved both in agitating for workers' rights but also forming a crucial locus of nationalist agitation against British rule.[19] While the union that was officially recognized after Independence, the RMMS, has remained affiliated with the Congress party and been generally accommodating of the changes faced by the textile industry and mill workers over the past decades, other unions more opposed to these changes became particularly active in the 1980s as the mill closures started in earnest.[20]

The event that in a sense both marked the moment of intensity of the trade union movement and anticipated its slow demise was the textile workers' strike of 1982, one of the major events in the recent history of Bombay. This was the largest strike in the history of Bombay, lasting for over a year and involving over 250,000 mill workers.[21] It was led by the charismatic and controversial union leader Datta Samant, who was assassinated in 1997, apparently by contract killers. The strike signified a strongly articulated moment of working class consciousness and solidarity, but also, in a sense, signified the crisis of deindustrialization that the mills were already facing.[22]

The dominant sociality is seen in the continued presence of mill workers' unions, which retain their sense of working class identity and solidarity, but without the sense of unified purpose that marked their heyday in the 1980s. A number of Samant's own campaigns in the 1990s ended in failure, leading to a questioning of his strategy and tactics amongst workers' groups. The crucial change in the actions of a union such as GKSS involves its shifting focus towards tenancy rights, highlighting the way in which *land* rather than *labor* has become the dominant locus of value.

What relevance does this engagement with labor and land issues on the part of workers movement in Bombay have to do with biosociality? One reading of the situation is that since the mill workers do not form social identifications based on shared biological identification, this case is not about biosociality. As Rabinow himself says in the Afterword to this volume, "[t]he term [biosociality] was not intended as a universal. It does not apply everywhere and at all times."

My interest in this essay is not to reiterate this obvious point. It is instead to ask the question of how biosociality *does* appear in the situation that I have described here. I believe that the situations concerning the loss of work and struggles over land tenancy speak to specific configurations of subjectivity within larger structures of capital that are of relevance in understanding the subject-constitutions of biocapital. In the instance of the mill districts, there is evidently a working *class* subjectivity, one consequent to the residual formation of industrial capital, but also one that is under threat of erasure. This is in part because labor is less and less the locus of struggle (making class antagonism a less self-evident structural locus of identification), but most directly because of a weakening of the unions, consequent to their own internal struggles, divisions and failures, and because part of the structural consequences of the evisceration of industry involves pushing more and more workers into informal sectors of work, and therefore away from trade unions.[23]

There is, second, strong emergent *consumer* subjectivity, corresponding to the dominant formation of speculative capital. This consumer subjectivity is reflected in the presence and actions of the middle class, which constitutes the potential market for the real estate developers who wish to build on the mill lands, and also constitutes the actual market for the many consumer goods that are sold in newly constructed shopping malls in the mill districts. An example of such a shopping mall is shown in the photograph. This is of Phoenix Mills, now referred to as "High Street Phoenix," one of the glitziest shopping malls in the mill districts, which has preserved the façade of the mill that once existed. In a sense, the transformation of Phoenix Mills to Phoenix Mall exemplifies the structural transformations that have happened in Bombay over the last two decades; the façade of the mill, however, is testament to the residual formation of industrial capital that still remains.[24] And third, there is the *experimental* subjectivity of the mill workers who get recruited into clinical trials – in its particulars, unique perhaps to Parel and Wellspring, but in its generalities, speaking to an entire nation of potential experimental subjects as clinical research capacity gets ramped up at a national level in anticipation of getting global trials.

What I am arguing for, in other words, is that there are at least three levels or registers of subjectivity – a working class subjectivity, a consumer subjectivity, and an experimental subjectivity – that exist in Bombay today, corresponding to the residual, dominant and emergent forms of industrial, speculative and bio-capital. This argument, in order to be fleshed out, begs two further questions:

1   Whenever one thinks of subjectivity in capitalism, one is confronted with the question of antagonism. Marx posed this question of irreducible antagonism between the worker and capital, and between the worker and the capitalist (not the same thing, and its mergers and distinctions are absolutely crucial to tease out) as a central part of his working through of the labor theory of value. While there are many who read this as an essentialist diagnosis that reduces politics to that of class, I wish to suggest, at least parenthetically, that Marx arrives at this diagnosis after a very careful and particular analysis of the contradictions inherent to the *money-form*. According to Marx, the multiple functions of money – as means of exchange, measure of exchange, and as universal equivalent – are internally contradictory with respect to each other in ways that

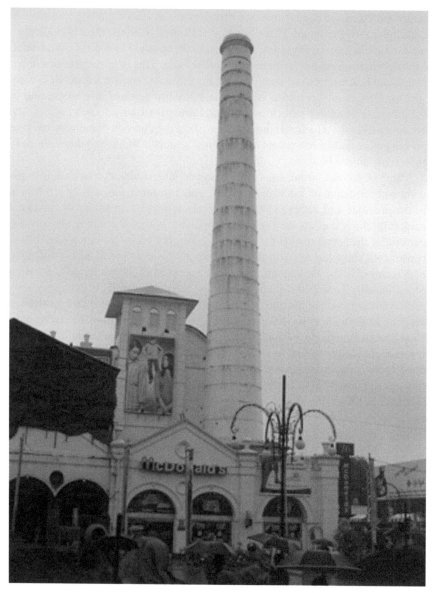

Figure 8.1 Phoenix Mills, now High Street Phoenix (photograph taken in July 2004)

anticipate social antagonism between those who can circulate it as capital and those who are subjected to it as wage.[25] Even if one does not buy the argument for a necessary antagonism in these various capital formations that coexist in Bombay, it is essential at the very least to ask whether such antagonism exists; what shape it takes in each of the residual, dominant and emergent capital forms that I have described here; and

who that antagonism is towards (if "capitalist," then what the subjectivity
and sociality of the capitalist in question might be).

2   If there are at least three distinct registers of subjectivity at stake here
     – of workers, consumers, and experimental subjects, each in a respec-
     tive relationship of production with mill owners, speculators and
     hospital owners – then under what circumstances might each of these
     subjectivities become *socialities*, transform into the locus of shared
     social identifications?

In answer to the first question, the "capitalists" here, as just mentioned, are
mill owners, real estate speculators, and hospital owners. Crucially, in the case of
Bombay, it is possible for these three groups to be virtually identical. For instance,
as mentioned earlier, Wellspring was seeded by NPIL, a national pharmaceutical
company run by the Piramal family. Crossroads, another large shopping mall
opened in Parel quite close to Wellspring, was also developed by the Piramals
and opened in 1999. And indeed, the Piramals have for decades been mill owners.
The Piramals are one of the largest industrial families in India, representing a
3.5 billion rupee conglomerate.[26] The Piramals therefore embody within a single
family business the residual, dominant and emergent formations of capital in
Bombay today.

I believe that this is not merely contingent, but follows a historical pattern
of family business strategy in India, and also has structural consequences. For
instance, many of the other big family businesses in India, such as Reliance
and Dabur, have started life science and pharmaceutical divisions, with clinical
research either already or likely to be a crucial component of these divisions (as
with the Piramals, Reliance initially started off in textiles, in the other center of
textile manufacturing in India, Ahmedabad). A third such business, Modi, is in the
process of starting a teaching university which will include a diploma certificate in
Clinical Research Management. In other words, there is an always already shared
social identification amongst the capitalists, in Bombay specifically but perhaps
more generally as well, which in the Indian case often has its locus in the family
business, but which occurs through a value generation that spans different epochal
manifestations of capitalism.

This is where the potential structural consequences lie. For in a sense, what I
have just pointed to are the conditions of possibility for a capitalist *class* to exist
in Bombay, consequent to the structural relations of production that are prevalent
there. Crucially, as structural transformation from industrial to speculative (and
bio-) capital occurs in Bombay, *there is no necessary disruption in this class
consciousness*, because the same players are dealing all three sets of cards. Indeed,
potential losses in one sector of capitalism (such as textiles) can be easily offset
by value accrued in another (such as real estate), to the extent that, as Isswalkar
pointed out, it is actually in the interests of mill owners that their mills shut down.

A similar congruence between subjectivity and actors' identities does not
however exist in the case of those impacted by these structural changes in
capitalism. The retrenched mill workers do not constitute the new consumer

class of Bombay. That is constituted primarily by those who work in the service industries – either members of an affluent middle class, or, indeed, young service workers in industries that do back-end contract work for Western corporations (such as call centers, back-end software technical support, back-end financial services, and the like) who come to cities from rural or small-town India in search of such work. Many of these service workers are in their early twenties, single, and earn up to three times as much as they would have done working, for instance, in a public sector steel industry, which would have been the likely profession they would have entered in an earlier generation.[27] Most of their wage ends up being disposable income, and these workers are very much a part of the consuming middle class population of cities like Bombay. The mill workers and experimental subjects, coincidentally and in some cases, end up being the same people, but in their latter subjectivity they are individuated, and not represented by the trade unions (or anyone else) *as experimental subjects*. To the extent that a *class consciousness* exists amongst any of these groups, it is amongst the workers. And that class consciousness, historically, came about not as an inevitable consequence of a structural subject position, but in large measure because of the community sensibility that built around the *chawls*, and because of decades of union organizing. It is a class consciousness that is under erasure as the *chawls* are threatened with demolition, as the organizing capacities of the unions become weaker, and as work becomes less and less the locus of political organization. Indeed, if a *structural subject position within relations of production* is the basis of shared social identity formation amongst the capitalists, then it is, in contrast, a *contingent political and urban history* that forms such a basis amongst the workers.

My argument here is that part of the way in which capital structures unequal power relations between those who control relations of production and those are subjected by it is by differentially configuring sociality in each case, whereby it is always harder to form a shared social identification for those *subjected to* capital than for those who are *agents of* it.

I have tried to make this argument empirically here, by showing the contingency of working class formation in Bombay historically – a situation that is, in a sense, tailor made to the creation of a situation of strong working class solidarity. Indeed, an interesting symptomatic reading of my interview with Isswalkar is that the term "working class" appears only once, though "workers" are referred to many times.[28] When Isswalkar did use "working class," he did so to designate a general term (what happens to the working class when you turn Bombay into a Hong Kong or a Singapore?), rather than as a specific description of the mill workers' sociality.

While the contingent subject-position of the working class in Bombay could be argued for from empirical ethnographic material (as I have done here), it could perhaps more generally be argued for as part of the *symptomatic structure* of capital. For indeed, Étienne Balibar points to the symptomatic absence of the word "proletariat" in Marx's later works dealing with the labor theory of value, except in the initial parts of the section of so-called primitive accumulation in

Volume 1 of *Capital*, where it is used in a specific historical register to refer to the proletarianization of labor as part of the process of industrialization in England.[29] Balibar shows, through this reading, that for Marx (or certainly for the Marx of *Capital*), the proletariat, or a working *class* with the shared social consciousness that constitutes such a formation, never exists consequent to structural relations of production. This produces an aporetic moment in Marx's philosophy, because the aim of the communist revolution that he hopes for is to destroy the existing class relations of capital; but for these class relations to be destroyed, the working class has to be called into existence first (organizationally and contingently), and a class consciousness has to be created that is *not* structural.

What is crucial here is the inverse of this argument, for Balibar also argues that in contrast, the capitalist *class* does exist structurally for Marx.[30] This is evidenced in Marx's transition, in Volume 1 of *Capital*, from an analysis of absolute to relative surplus value. The analysis of absolute surplus value forms the theoretical core of the labor theory of value; it is in surplus value that Marx identifies the locus of exploitation of the worker in capitalism. This is because the wage that the worker receives is always *inadequate* to the work he can (potentially) perform; this inadequacy is the measure of surplus value, and the measure of exploitation.

But absolute surplus value is a purely *hypothetical* construct. It is, for Marx, a schematic rendering of the interactions between a single capitalist and a single worker. A more empirical rendering of these interactions as they take place is suggested by his notion of *relative* surplus value, which is the value that is accrued in the interaction between a group of capitalists and a group of workers. And here, Marx suggests that surplus value is not a measure that can be calculated in individuated fashion for each capitalist, but is rather an *aggregate potentiality*, a potential value generation over and above wage expenditure that operates to increase the value of capital writ large. In other words, surplus value functions in a way that leads to the structural cohesion of individual interests of capitalists into the collective interest of capital. It is thus that the subjectivity of the capitalist is always already predisposed to being a shared social identification.

For Marx, therefore, the worker and the capitalist might be antagonistic subjectivities, but the working class and the capitalist class are not equivalent socialities. The conditions of possibility for the existence of each are asymmetrical. One sees empirical manifestations of this in Bombay. There is a seamless convergence between the interests of mill owners and real estate speculators (not least because they are oftentimes the same people); there is no such seamless convergence amongst the workers. Let alone between mill workers and service workers – even for unemployed mill workers, as Isswalkar anxiously diagnosed at a number of points in our conversation, the default subject-position, in the absence of union organizing, is either lumpenization in the case of younger people (joining the underworld and becoming a gangster), or suicide in the case of older ones. In other words, for the workers, the structurally formed subject-position in Bombay is not one of shared social identification, but rather one of desperate individuation and alienation.

In the relationship between capitalist and industrial/factory worker, money is the locus around which differentially contingent socialities take shape. This is because for the worker, money is adequated as wage; but for the capitalist, that wage is exchanged for labor power, which is the potential for labor over and above that remunerated in wage, and therefore surplus. In this way, while money is wage for the worker, it is capital for the capitalist. The methodological question is whether a similar analytic as that which Marx applies to elucidating the relationship between capitalist value and the formation of differential socialities can be applied to biosociality. Conceptually, this question can be rearticulated as – what recalibrations in value and subjectivity occur in biosociality that allow shared identity formations to emerge (compared, for instance, to those that prevailed in industrial capitalism)?

I believe that an answer to such a question cannot be attempted except by historicizing biocapital against other/earlier structural formations of capital. This can easily be done in Bombay because of the coexistence of biocapitalist formations with those of industrial and speculative capitalism. If one considers the residual formation of the closing textile mills, money and (wage-) labor become the focal points of differential sociality (the interests of the capitalist mill owners pitted against those of unemployed workers, who get represented as a working class by the trade union movement). This is specific to the story of the mill districts of Bombay, but shows the general structural features of capitalist antagonism that Marx diagnosed a century and a half ago. If one considers the dominant formation of the boom in speculative real estate, it is land and tenancy that become the focal points of differential sociality (the interests of the capitalist real estate speculators pitted against those of the *chawl* dwellers who will have no place to live once their tenements are torn down). This too is specific to the mill districts – indeed, the *chawls* are a unique part of the local architecture – but one sees this question of tenancy as an emergent locus of worker/community mobilization as a consistent theme in other parts of the world as well.[31]

If one considers the emergent form of biocapital (crucial components of which, as argued earlier in this essay, are genomics and clinical trials) then it is scientific knowledge combined with consumption capabilities that become the focal points of differential sociality. In other words – while biosocial subjects are evidently formed consequent to biomedical epistemology, the biosociality that Rabinow imagines in terms of efficiency, adaptability and the capacity for self-fashioning is meaningless unless one recognizes that these emergent biosocial subjects are also *consumers*; consumers of biomedical technology and epistemology, but also, given the dominant mode of production of such technology and epistemology today, consumers on the *market*. Further, the diagnostic capabilities of biomedicine that form the immediate conditions of possibility for biosociality to take shape are themselves a stabilized consequence of earlier *experimental* procedures (whether in the laboratory, on animals, or on humans), which means that experimentation is a constitutive element of this form of life that emerges consequent to knowledge – consumption assemblages.

This begs the question of where the experimental subject fits in to a political economy of biocapital, and what such a subject-position has to do with the efficient, adaptable and self-fashioning biosociality that Rabinow anticipates in his essay. For that, one has to return to the question of what the locus of subjectivity is in the case of biocapital. If it is labor in the case of industrial capital, and land in the case of speculative capital (in Bombay at least), then it is, as suggested earlier in this essay, *health* (articulated through a *risk* calculus) in the case of biocapital.

Just as labor means different things for the different people implicated in the political economy of industrial capital (work performed in exchange for wage for the worker; labor power for the capitalist); or land means different things in the political economy of real estate (a place to live for the tenant; a financial investment and locus of future appreciating value for the owner of the land); so too does risk have different meanings within the political economy of biomedicine. For the biosocial subject that Rabinow anticipates, risk is an epistemology of self-fashioning (as already suggested). It is a risk that is predicated on free consumer choice, but indeed is in itself deeply subjugating. The risk logic that Rabinow describes plays out on the one hand as agential formations based on shared biological identifications (seen most evidently as patient advocacy groups), but on the other hand plays out as an interpellation to prophylactic behavior – a responsible subject, within this risk logic, would not just organize after the fact of disease, but indeed embrace preventive measures that would negate the onset of potential illness in the first place. Crucially, preventive medicine increasingly includes within its constitutive ambit the consumption of therapeutics, including therapeutics that were initially developed as cures for diseases, but are increasingly marketed as "chronic" necessities. Disease risk as an epistemology of self-fashioning, in addition to being biosocial, also subjects individuals to potentially perpetual therapeutic consumption, turning them into always already patients-in-waiting.[32]

The second register at which I argued risk functions (drawing on François Ewald) is as capital. This is the register at which it functions for the biotechnology and pharmaceutical industries. Disease risk foretold by biomedical technologies and epistemologies creates a potential market for diagnostic and therapeutic consumption, and this constitutes a crucial source of market value for drug companies.

One already sees in place here a structure of antagonism, in this case between the market producers of therapy (and diagnostics) and potentially biosocial consumers, which in crucial respects mirrors that between worker and capitalist, and this is the parallel that Joseph Dumit develops in his forthcoming book *Drugs for Life*. Here, the exploitation is not at the level of surplus value, but of what Dumit calls surplus health – the capacity for therapeutic consumption over and above that required to combat disease.

Before going on to thinking about risk in its third register, as labor, I wish to mark here the crucial epochal transition between industrial and biocapital that a notion such as biosociality marks. While there are many uncanny parallels between the risk logics of surplus health and the labor logics of surplus value, there is also a crucial difference, and this is, as Dumit puts it, a transition of the biomedical industry from being "an arm of capital (charged with maintaining workers for work)" to becoming "an industry itself" (Dumit 2004). In other words, what is at stake here is not the maintenance of health for *work's* sake (the reproduction of the conditions of production through a reproduction of labor power by keeping the worker healthy, which was the logic of health within industrial capital), but for *health's* sake – health itself becomes the source of value, it does not have to be materialized in labor for it to become valuable.

The exception is the experimental subjects' labor, which is constituted by their subjection to the risk of clinical experimentation as a condition of possibility for the sorts of therapeutic development that the logic of surplus health depends upon. I wish to elaborate upon this figure in the next section, by moving away from the specific case of the mill workers of Bombay to look at a more generalized emergence of experimental subjectivity in India consequent to a ramping up of clinical research capacity there. I therefore juxtapose my story of Bombay to that of one of India's oldest and most established CROs, Vimta Laboratories, located in Hyderabad.

V

It could be called Foucault Street. It is in the middle of nowhere, one of the many urban peripheries outside Hyderabad that have recently developed as technoscientific satellite cities. It is a dusty street, just like any other dusty street leading out of Hyderabad. At the start of the dusty street is an asylum, next to which is a high-tech prison. Towards the end of the street is the dark grey edifice of Vimta, one of the oldest and arguably the most aggressively growing and business savvy clinical research organization (CRO) in India today.

I am transported through this company on a tour. I start in the corporate offices, where I am met by the company's director of clinical research. She takes me to her office and gives me the obligatory Power Point presentation. I am then walked through the clinical trials assembly line as it is set up. There is the waiting and screening room, which looks like the waiting room of a railway station, where trial subjects come in and are given their consent forms and a basic questionnaire to fill out in order to determine whether they are qualified to participate in the trial. The walls of the waiting room are empty, except for a single bulletin board that outlines all the risks that could accrue to participants who are in a clinical trial. The only language that the board is written in is English. I am told that in order to participate in a trial, the subjects have to be literate (though not necessarily in English), and they are invariably male (Vimta only enrolls females if the trial sponsor specifies a need for female subjects).

After the waiting room is a long corridor, with many rooms where different types of medical examinations are conducted on trial volunteers. First, their height and weight are recorded. If the subject is less than 55 kg, he is not admitted into the trial because the risk of trial-related complications becomes too high. There is then a general physical exam, after which the tests become progressively more invasive – an ECG is conducted in a third room, blood drawn in a fourth (which is sent to the pathology labs for analysis), and an X-ray taken in a fifth. I learn while being walked through this corridor that the consent forms the subjects sign in the waiting room are specifically for the medical screening procedures – if they are selected to participate in the trial, they sign a separate form, which is particular to the trial they are enrolled on. A number of the trials conducted at Vimta are Phase I trials on healthy volunteers. Recruiting subjects into Phase I trials has become increasingly difficult in the United States, which is one of the stated rationalities for taking these trials to other countries (these are much less expensive than Phase III trials, so it is ease of recruitment rather than cost that forms the most compelling rationale for their globalization). I am told that volunteer retention is much better in India than in the US, because "people trust doctors here." I am intrigued that while recruiting healthy people to have risky molecules administered to them is such a challenge, the entire set-up seems to emphasize "selection" – it is almost as if getting enrolled into a trial is a test that only those who are fit enough can pass. I am also intrigued that the subjects are only ever referred to as "volunteers," suggesting no doubt their autonomous rational agency, the same agency that gets contractually codified through the consent form. As we walk through the corridors, I ask how volunteer recruitment occurs. I am told that it is mainly by posting advertisements in the local newspapers. Can I get a copy of such an ad from them, I wonder? I am told I cannot, for proprietary reasons. I wonder why and how something that is in the public domain, like a newspaper ad, is deemed too "proprietary" to share with me, while it is perfectly alright for me to walk through the innards of the CRO taking notes on what I see, when the company knows that my purpose in doing so is to write about it. I shrug in perplexity, smile sheepishly, and walk on.

I next encounter the Phase I units where the clinical trials are performed. These are rooms with rows and rows of hospital beds. Three such rooms are completely empty, because no trials are being conducted in them. The fourth is full of study subjects, about thirty of them. They are doing nothing except lying in bed. All of them are in identical green hospital clothing. Some of them are watching the solitary TV screen at the far end of the room. One of them is looking at his watch. A few are asleep. Most are just staring vacantly into space. While all of these are apparently literate subjects, not one of them is reading – not even a newspaper or a magazine, which normally get read and discussed on every street corner in India, constantly. I of course am not allowed to talk to these trial "volunteers," or determine their identity. There is a male doctor at the table in the front of a room, stacks of files with patient records on the desk in front of him. His assistant, female, is sitting on an adjacent stool, which is appropriately shorter than his chair, entering data into the records.

The next room, at the time darkened and secluded, only has four beds in it. This, I am told, is the intensive care unit where patients are admitted and administered to in case of adverse events during a trial. It suddenly brings home to me the nature of this high-risk activity. It looks like a medical emergency room that might exist in a factory to attend to accidents on the factory floor. It re-emphasizes not just that experimental subjectivity is high-risk, but that it is, specifically, high-risk *labor*.

In his Afterword to this volume, Rabinow refers to the linking of different "domains of practice" by the concept biosociality. These include, in his articulation, "genomics, pastoral care, patients' rights, alliance with researchers, etc." The situation at Vimta figures as the "etc." – while genomic experiments might be performed in such a set-up, these subjects are not patients (except in the case of an adverse event, when they would become one in the ICU), they are in no way allied with the researchers, and this is absolutely not about pastoral care, certainly not for those physically present and experimented upon within those walls.

And yet, they are participating in an enterprise that absolutely *is* about pastoral care. To take Dumit's epochal diagnosis further, if the instrumental logic of industrial capital (health for work's sake) becomes a self-perpetuating logic in biocapital (health for health's sake) when one considers logics of therapeutic consumption, then inversely, the self-perpetuating logic of industrial capital (work for work's sake, the logic to which the employed mill worker in Parel, for instance, is subjected) becomes the instrumental logic of biocapital (work for health's sake, the logic to which the experimental subject – whether at Vimta, or perhaps an unemployed mill worker in Parel – is subjected).

It is because such experimental subjects are outside the circuits of pastoral care (and therapeutic consumption) that they come to be "merely risked." But the crucial point I wish to make is that the very circuits of pastoral care and therapeutic consumption that these subjects fall out of *can only be constituted in the first place through the existence of such "merely risked" subjects*. These experimental subjects provide the conditions of possibility for the neo-liberal consumer subjects who generate surplus health, or for the neo-liberal biosocial subjects who form shared social identifications in the cause of patient advocacy.

The figure of the merely risked experimental subject, in my mind, is structurally parallel to the figure of the subaltern that Gayatri Spivak writes about in her critique of Foucault and Deleuze (Spivak 1988). The subaltern, for Spivak, does not refer to some general nebulous notion of the oppressed or structurally less well off subject. It is a *specific* subject formed consequent to specific social relations – in her case, of labor, gender and colonial histories. An exemplary subaltern figure, therefore, is the woman who commits *sati*, whose subjectivity comes to be only at the moment of her death, of a "voluntary" suicide that she is forced to commit upon her husband's death. A second, developed in subsequent work, is that of the Third World female home-worker – subjected simultaneously to histories of capitalism and colonialism that see the outsourcing of labor to parts of the world where it is cheapest to perform; of gender inequities that differentially structure wage and organizational capacities; and of an *informalization* of labor in which certain essential types of work become invisible. Crucially, Spivak argues that such informal labor is absolutely essential to the constitution of global capital (Spivak 1999).

While the experimental subject, I argue, is a condition of possibility for biosociality and the neo-liberal therapeutic consumer, there is an additional point that I wish to make, which is the *structural impossibility* of such a figure being a *political* subject. This does not mean that experimental subjects cannot politically mobilize; there are many conditions under which they conceivably could. But those conditions would be purely contingent, and one of the contingencies that would most likely lead to a political subjectivity for these subjects (either organized or otherwise) would be through pain and/or death, for instance through a likely scandal that would result from a serious adverse event in a Phase I clinical trial.[33] The biosocial subject that Rabinow conceives of is almost by definition in the realm of articulatory politics (articulation here referring both to the capacity of having a political voice, and of forming sociopolitical linkages).[34] The experimental subject, like Spivak's subaltern figure, is on the other hand, in her evocative metaphor, in shadow.

The way in which the experimental subject *does* get figured is *ethically*. And the ethical figuration occurs through informed consent. Certainly in the Indian situations that I have encountered, whether at Wellspring or at Vimta, there is a serious and absolute concern with adequate informed consent procedures. There is a concerted effort led by the Indian state and driven by Indian CROs to build a robust ethical infrastructure to regulate clinical research, including a nation-wide system of institutional review boards. Indian clinical researchers bristle at the aspersion that global clinical trials come to India because it is easier to cut corners there. Indeed, the Indian government in 2005 passed a series of laws, called Schedule Y, to insist upon good clinical practice (which primarily involves strong regulatory oversight on clinical research combined with proper procedures for collecting informed consent). The Indian laws are the only ones in the world which deem the violation of good clinical practice to be a criminal rather than a civil offense. Explicit attention is given to the fact that many trial subjects in an Indian context are likely to be illiterate; questions of how proper informed consent can be obtained in such situations are attended to deeply.[35]

Adriana Petryna diagnoses that "'ethics' [gets] configured ... to justify a massive expansion of commercialized human subjects research" (Petryna 2005b). I wish to further this assessment by suggesting that ethics does not just *legitimate* experimental subjectivity, it actively *depoliticizes* it. Petryna further argues for a state of "ethical variability" in global clinical trials, suggesting that ethical rationales, commercial imperatives and the modes of conduct of these trials eventually lead to differential ethical standards applied in different parts of the world (with the Third World invariably being the site of greater laxity) (Petryna 2005a, 2005b). While I am generally persuaded by Petryna's argument, the ethical variability in India's case is, if anything, one of *hyperethicality*. Vimta is an exemplary site for me not because it is a scandalous example of dubious trial practices, but because it is in many ways the gold standard for CROs to aspire to. It is one of the oldest CROs in India, established as far back as 1992. It is the only Indian CRO to be publicly traded on the national stock market, making it accountable to public investors. It is the only Indian CRO to have been audited twice by the US Food and Drug Administration (FDA), passing both with flying colors. The manager of clinical research at a US-based company, looking for Indian collaborators, indicated to me that Vimta would be the ideal sort of company from her perspective to collaborate with, not just because they possess the infrastructure for the conduct of clinical research, but because she felt comfortable with their ethical practices.

The violence of experimental subjectivity in the case of Parel might be exacerbated by the particular historical conjuncture of the mill districts. But as my superimposed account of Vimta hopefully shows, the violence of such subjectivity is not contingent or scandalous but rather structural. And it is a structural violence without which biosociality, as it has taken shape within neo-liberal logics of consumption, would be inconceivable.

VI

Étienne Balibar suggests a dual meaning for the term *critique*, suggesting "on the one hand, the eradication of error; on the other, knowledge on the limits of a faculty or practice" (Balibar 1996: 18). It is in this sense that I have attempted to critique biosociality in this essay, by probing at the limits of the concept. Rabinow himself suggests a concern with the limits of this concept in his Afterword. He says:

> By the turn of the century, however, some of the limits of the concept could now be seen with more clarity. The identification of such limitations is most welcome as biosociality was intended as a concept and not as an epochal designation ... that is to say, the term did not have the same analytic power everywhere ... Inquiry reveals specificities and limits, an excellent definition of critical thinking.

But my meaning of "limit" here is two-fold – it means that outside of which biosociality cannot exist (limit as *boundary*), but equally that which constitutes the threshold condition for biosociality, *without* which it cannot exist. My speculation here is that the experimental subject forms the limiting figure for biosociality, but in *both* of these senses.

The care with which Rabinow has used biosociality – as a concept rather than an epochal designation – is precisely, in my mind, the reason that it has been such a promissory and generative concept. It is one that has attempted not to close down critical thought by making a pronouncement about an era or a regime, but has rather emphasized and performed the open-endedness of a set of emergent phenomena that have crucial consequences for our calibrations of life, labor and language, for our understandings of what "the social" might mean. More specifically, it functions as a diagnostic probe into a particular set of discourses and practices as they unfold at a particular moment in time.

In this essay, I have attempted to flesh out this diagnostic and anticipatory move that Rabinow makes with the concept of biosociality by turning instead to Michael Fischer's heuristic of "emergent forms of life" (Fischer 2003). This is a shift in methodological accent away from a concern with the likely contours of emergent phenomena (a mapping exercise, which was also Foucault's method of teasing out the components of modernity, or society, or life itself), towards a concern with the question of how particular socialities of action *come to be*. The comparison here is a concern with *form*, on the one hand (Rabinow) and that of *process*, on the other (Fischer). My suggestion here is that the limits of a concept can only be probed by a working through of how that concept *comes to be* in particular times and places. In this sense, it is impossible to disentangle critique from questions of method.

What this means for me, in part, is the impossibility of a seamless narrative. On the one hand, this story is "about" the mill workers-turned-experimental subjects of Parel. The particular historical conjunctures within which the story of Parel is situated are absolutely crucial, and it is the function of ethnography to delineate these particularities. At the same time, on the other hand, this story is not about Parel at all. It can only make sense if unbounded from its locality (in other words, even if Parel's particular histories are crucial, Parel itself is always already a local, trans-local and global site. It is a particular community with its own historically evolved sociality; it is emblematic of the urban character of Bombay as an emergent "global city";[36] it has been and continues to be a transnational node in the flow of various forms of capital, industrial, speculative and bio). And truly contextualizing Parel involves looking to other sites at which clinical research is happening (Vimta in Hyderabad, for instance, but also other parts of the world); other sites at which worker and community mobilization is happening around tenancy rights (Alexandria, perhaps, or Cape Town); or other places where the textile industry has been eviscerated, something that I have not done in this essay.[37]

Similarly, this is a story that needs to be unbounded in time, and looked at not just as a particular contingent event (concerning retrenchment, clinical infrastructure building, and experimental subject-formation), but in terms of multiple structural horizons. It needs to be attentive to the epistemic fluidities that are involved in the formation of subjectivities and socialities, which in the case of the mill workers of Parel take shape consequent to the role of cytochrome P-450 enzymes in oxidative drug metabolism as much as they do because of colonial histories and political economic logics of the textile industry. And finally, it is a story that needs to be unbounded conceptually, so that while it is "about" the figure of the experimental subject, it is approached from a whole range of situated perspectives that are not those of experimental subjects at all. Indeed, the one set of actors who do not directly figure as ethnographic actors in this essay are the experimental subjects themselves, not least because the ethical apparatus of clinical research makes them the most difficult actors to access. In this sense, I have in this essay shadowed the experimental subject – followed him around, even to his hospital bed, but also failed (structurally rather than intentionally) to give him voice.[38]

It is this lack of seamlessness that I feel is constitutive to the performance of George Marcus and Michael Fischer's call for multi-sited ethnography, a sensibility that points to the methodological impossibility of tracing emergent global phenomena without understanding the complex topologies – historical, spatial and scalar – that they inhabit.[39] Genomics, advanced liberalism, patient advocacy – those are the frameworks within which biosociality functions smoothly. My interest in this essay has been instead to critique biosociality by exploring its limits, and highlighting its striations.

Acknowledgements

I would like to thank Joseph Dumit, Michael Fisher, Sahra Gibbon, Carlos Novas, Kristin Peterson, Rajeswari Sunder Rajan and Travis Tanner for invaluable comments on drafts of this manuscript.

Notes

1 See Sunder Rajan 2005 for an elaboration of this story.
2 For more about CBT, India's flagship public sector genome lab, see Sunder Rajan 2006.
3 In fact, pharmacogenomics is a double-edged sword for biotech and pharmaceutical companies from the perspective of value generation. This is because patient stratification based on drug efficacy is not necessarily a good thing for them, as it will likely result in market segmentation. (In other words, if you are a drug company, you really do not want your potential market to be restricted to those who will respond best to the drug.) On the other hand, patient stratification based on safety could be very valuable, because currently drugs are pulled off market altogether because a small segment of the population shows an adverse response to it. If that population segment could be genetically delineated, it might be possible to market the drug to the remaining population of "safe" responders instead of recalling the drug altogether.
4 For proprietary reasons, it is hard for me to access the exact list of corporate clients that Wellquest and Genomed has or had. Regardless of this, it is clear that getting global clinical trials contracts is part of the business model of Wellquest, and global pharmacogenomic research studies were definitely courted by Genomed.
5 For analyses of the evisceration of the textile industry in Bombay, see D'Monte 2002, Breman and Shah 2003, Breman 2004, Menon and Adarkar 2005.
6 This dual conception of subjectivity, as always already *subjected to* and *agent of*, is Hegelian. See Hegel 1979, and Balibar 1995 for an elaboration of this dialectic.
7 Rabinow 1996: 100.
8 Ibid.
9 See for instance Castel 1991. See also Dumit 1998.
10 For elaborations of risk-as-capital in the context of drug development, see Joe Dumit's forthcoming book *Drugs for Life*, and the conclusion to my book *Biocapital* (Sunder Rajan 2006).
11 While these industry figures are almost certainly exaggerated, as argued by Love 1997, 2001a, b, there is no question that drug development is a high-risk capital intensive process, with much of the risk and capital expenditure borne during clinical trials.
12 For an elaboration of this, see Chapter 4 of *Biocapital* (Sunder Rajan 2006).
13 For work that traces various elements of these, see Fisher 2005, Kuo 2005, Petryna 2005a, 2005b.
14 The other union is the Rashtriya Mill Mazdoor Sangh (National Mill Workers' Union, RMMS), which is officially affiliated to the Congress Party. The Congress has been one of the two major political parties that has ruled the state of Maharashtra, of which Bombay is capital, for the last three decades (the other being an alliance of the right-wing nationalist Bharatiya Janata Party (BJP) and the even more right-wing Shiv Sena, whose political platform is based on a highly exclusionary Maharashtrian

identity politics). Both the Congress and the BJP-Shiv Sena have political interests in shutting down the mills, not least because of close links to mill owners and real estate developers. The RMMS, consequently, has consistently advocated a more conciliatory approach towards mill owners, and has often been seen to abandon the causes of the mill workers.

15 The interview cited below was originally conducted in Hindi. I provide here my own English translation of it.

16 Emphasis on "working class" is my own, and I will return to this emphasis subsequently. For an account of middle-class sentiment towards, and state violence against, hawkers in Bombay today, see Rajagopal 2004.

17 Indeed, two of the most notorious gangs in Bombay in the 1990s were led by Arun Gawli and Sudhir Naik, both sons of mill-workers.

18 It is generally difficult to find out who gets recruited into clinical trials, in part because the process of recruitment itself provides protection to the trial subjects' privacy by providing them with anonymity. Kris Peterson's work in Nigeria is an exciting exception, as she has managed to trace down a number of people who were on experimental anti-retroviral trials conducted there in the mid-1990s, and has been interviewing them in an attempt to reconstruct the trial from the perspective of the experimental subjects.

19 The nationalism of the mill workers was often at odds with the mainstream nationalist movement represented by the Indian National Congress, largely because it was more militant. In the 1940s, for instance, mill workers' movements aligned themselves with Subash Chandra Bose, who had broken ranks with the Congress in his opposition to Gandhi's non-violent strategies, and in his desire to ally with the Japanese against the British in World War II.

20 See note 14 for RMMS.

21 For historical overviews of the strike, see Omvedt 1983, Bakshi 1986, Lakha 1988, van Wersch 1992.

22 Historically, this could be said to be the second crisis of deindustrialization facing the Indian textile industry. The first occurred in the late nineteenth and early twentieth centuries, the crisis then being faced by handloom weavers in the face of competition from textiles that were being exported into India from the British mills by the colonial state. This eventually led to the establishment of mills in Indian cities (mainly Bombay and Ahmedabad), which were owned by British industrialists until independence, when they were nationalized. By the 1970s, many of the nationalized mills had been turned over to private Indian mill owners. If the first crisis of deindustrialization was caused by global circuits of capital controlled by colonial interests, then the second crisis could be said to be caused by global circuits of capital dictated by logics of neo-liberal, speculative finance. For a historical account of the Indian handloom industry through the twentieth century, see Roy 1993.

23 See Breman and Shah 2003 for an elaboration of this argument in the context of Ahmedabad.

24 Shekhar Krishnan wrote an excellent report for GRHS on the violent history of the shutting down of Phoenix Mills. See Krishnan 2000.

25 This is the argument with which Marx starts the *Grundrisse* (Marx 1973 [1858]). Crucially, he starts his analysis in Volume 1 of *Capital* with the *commodity* form, which is not irreducibly antagonistic, but rather fetishistic (Marx 1976 [1867]). In other words, the social antagonism that resides within money is irreducible, but that which resides within the commodity is veiled. I make this distinction here, because I think it is crucial to teasing out in careful fashion the different ways in which formations of capital lead to configurations of subjectivity, and to potential and actual forms of shared social identification.

26 The Piramals textile business started in 1934 when they took over the Morarjee Goculdas mills, one of the oldest textile mills in the country. Their foray into pharmaceuticals

occurred in 1988, when they acquired Nicholas Laboratories from Sara Lee to form NPIL. In 1993, they acquired a 74 percent stake in the Indian unit of Hoffmann-la Roche, and bought up Boehringer Mannheim India and the research division of Rhone Poulenc India. NPIL is now the fourth largest pharmaceutical company in India. In addition to Crossroads, the Piramals are developers of a corporate park in Lower Parel.

27 For a glorified and celebratory analysis of this type of service work, which focuses precisely on the relatively high wages in the service sector, see Das 2003. For an alternative viewpoint that posits such back-end work as exploitative outsourcing of work for lower wages than what would have to be paid to Western workers, see Trivedi 2003.

28 I did not quote the interview in its entirety, but at no other point in the interview did Isswalkar use the term "working class."

29 Balibar 1994. This mode of "symptomatic reading" is central to the method of Balibar and Louis Althusser, and refers to a mode of reading that looks for absences and elisions as marking the site of contradiction and aporia in philosophical texts – and therefore also, invariably, marking the site of productive philosophical critique. For an employment of this method to a reading of *Capital*, see Althusser and Balibar 1971.

30 Étienne Balibar, personal conversations. I am grateful to Balibar for these conversations, which have helped greatly in the development of my argument in this section.

31 I am particularly indebted to the work of, and conversations with, Dan Moshenberg here. Moshenberg is involved with the Washington DC based chapter of the Tenants and Workers Support Community (TWSC), which is involved in fighting for community rights amongst local (invariably immigrant, largely unorganized, sometimes undocumented) workers in the greater Washington DC area. The particular stories of workers in Alexandria, VA, where much of Moshenberg's work is performed, are very different from those of Parel, but the structural contours are uncannily similar. Alexandria was a predominantly working class neighborhood that has become progressively gentrified, a stated (and state) rationality being "security" (because of the proximity of Alexandria to the Pentagon). The gentrification of Alexandria has been particularly intense in the five years since the 9-11 attacks on the Pentagon, and has led to a spike in land prices, a rash of real estate speculation, and the displacement of these workers (many of whom are janitors or day laborers in DC) to the suburban peripheries of the DC metropolitan area. The locus of TWSC's struggle, therefore, is very much around tenancy rights. One can therefore imagine a structural diagram consisting in Bombay of GKSS : unemployed mill workers (many originally from other parts of India); real estate speculation in the context of neo-liberal urban development as corresponding to one in DC of TWSC; unorganized day laborers (many originally from various parts of Central America); real estate speculation in the context of the neo-liberal security state.

Moshenberg is also involved in similar community organizing of workers around tenancy issues in Cape Town, South Africa. I am grateful to Moshenberg, not just for sharing his accounts of activism with TWSC and in Cape Town with me, but also for his deep engagement with Marx's method, which has been a source of great education for me. Thanks also to Jon Liss of TWSC for conversations about the Committee and explanations of some of the structural and particular situations faced by workers in the DC area.

32 For an elaboration of this, see Dumit 2004 and forthcoming.

33 For a parallel analysis that argues for the subject of *sati* as only coming into being as a body in pain and dying, on the funeral pyre of her husband, see R. Sunder Rajan 1993.

34 Stuart Hall elaborates upon this dual meaning of articulation. See Grossberg 1996.

35 I make these assertions based on conversations with most of the individuals involved in establishing the regulatory and ethical infrastructure of clinical research in India,

and based on fieldwork at a workshop in Delhi at which regulatory guidelines were devised and standardized in consonance with national laws and international guidelines in February 2006.

36 See Sassen 2000 for an elucidation of "global cities."
37 In my mind, an ideal juxtaposition here would be to North Carolina's eviscerated textile industry, especially given that the Research Triangle Park there is one of the three hubs of clinical research in the United States (the other two being New Jersey and the Austin–San Antonio area in Texas).
38 Indeed, I am generally suspicious of a certain heroic ethnographic conceit that positions the anthropologist as the romantic savior of the native or subaltern voice.
39 See Marcus and Fischer 1986, Marcus 1998.

References

Althusser, Louis and Etienne Balibar (1998 [1971]) *Reading Capital*. New York, London: Verso.

Bakshi, Rajni (1986) *The Long Haul: The Historic Bombay Textile Strike*. Bombay: Build Documentation Centre.

Balibar, Étienne (1994) *Masses, Classes, Ideas: Studies of Politics and Philosophy Before and After Marx*. New York and London: Routledge.

Balibar, Étienne (1995) "The Infinite Contradiction," (trans) J.-M. Poisson, J. Lezra, *Yale French Studies* 88, 142–64.

Balibar, Étienne (1996) *The Philosophy of Marx*. New York and London: Verso.

Beck, Ulrich (1986) *Risk Society: Towards a New Modernity*. London: Sage Publications.

Breman, Jan (2004) *The Labouring Poor in India: Patterns of Exploitation, Subordination, and Exclusion*. Delhi: Oxford University Press.

Breman, Jan and Parthiv Shah (2003) *Working in the Mill No More*. Amsterdam: Amsterdam University Press.

Castel, Robert (1991) "From Dangerousness to Risk," in G. Burchell, C. Gordon and P. Miller (eds) *The Foucault Effect: Studies in Governmentality*. Chicago, IL: University of Chicago Press.

Collier, Stephen and Andrew Lakoff (2005) "On Regimes of Living," in A. Ong and S. Collier (eds) *Global Assemblages: Technology, Politics, and Ethics as Anthropological Problems*. Malden, MA: Blackwell.

D'Monte, Darryl (2002) *Ripping the Fabric: The Decline of Mumbai and its Mills*. Delhi: Oxford University Press.

Das, Gurcharan (2003) "Cyber coolies or cyber sahibs?" *Times of India*, 7 September.

DiMasi, J.A., Hansen, R.W., Grabowski, H.G. and Lasagna, L. (1991) "Cost of Innovation in the Pharmaceutical Industry," *Journal of Health Economics*, July: 107–42.

Dumit, Joseph (1998) "A Digital Image of the Category of the Person: PET Scanning and Objective Self-Fashioning," in G. Downey and J. Dumit (eds) *Cyborgs and Citadels: Anthropological Interventions in Emerging Sciences and Technologies*. Santa Fe, NM: School of American Research.

Dumit, Joseph (2004) "Drugs, Algorithms, Markets and Surplus Health." Workshop paper presented at Department of Anthropology, University of California, Irvine.

Dumit, Joseph (forthcoming) *Drugs for Life*. Durham, NC: Duke University Press.

Ewald, François (1991) "Insurance and Risk," in G. Burchell, C. Gordon, and P. Miller (eds) *The Foucault Effect: Studies in Governmentality*. Chicago, IL: University of Chicago Press.

Fischer, Michael M.J. (2003) *Emergent Forms of Life and the Anthropological Voice.* Durham, NC: Duke University Press.

Fisher, Jill (2005) "Human Subjects in Medical Experiments," in S. Restivo (ed.) *Science, Technology, and Society.* New York: Oxford University Press.

Foucault, Michel (1990 [1978]) *The History of Sexuality: An Introduction.* New York: Vintage Books.

Grossberg, Lawrence (1996) "On Postmodernism and Articulation: an Interview with Stuart Hall," in D. Morley and K.-H. Chen (eds) *Stuart Hall: Critical Dialogues in Cultural Studies.* London and New York: Routledge.

Hegel, Georg Wilhelm Friedrich (1979) *Phenomenology of Spirit.* New York: Oxford University Press.

Krishnan, Shekhar (2000) "The Murder of the Mills: A Case Study of Phoenix Mills." Report by the Girangaon Bachao Andolan and Lokshahi Hakk Sanghatana.

Kuo, Wen-Hua (2005) "Japan and Taiwan in the Wake of Bio-Globalization: Drugs, Race, and Standards." PhD dissertation in the History and Social Studies of Science and Technology, Massachusetts Institute of Technology.

Lakha, Salim (1988) "Organized Labor and Militant Unionism: The Bombay Textile Workers' Strike of 1982," *Bulletin of Concerned Asian Scholars*, 20: 42.

Love, James (1997) "Calls for More Reliable Costs Data on Clinical Trials," *Marketletter*, 13 January: 24–5.

Love, James (2001a) "CPTech Release on Tufts Study and IRS Data" [online]. Available at: http://lists/essential.org/pipermail.ip-health/2001-November/002481.html.

Love, James (2001b) "Reporting on $802 Number – Clinical Trials Costs" [online]. Available at: http://lists.essential.org/pipermail/ip-health/2001-December/002484.html.

Marcus, George (1998) *Ethnography Through Thick and Thin.* Princeton, NJ: Princeton University Press.

Marcus, George and Michael M.J. Fischer (1986) *Anthropology as Cultural Critique: An Experimental Moment in the Human Sciences.* Chicago, IL: University of Chicago Press.

Marx, Karl (1973 [1858]) *Grundrisse: Foundations of the Critique of Political Economy.* Trans. Martin Nicolaus. London: Penguin Books.

Marx, Karl (1976 [1867]) *Capital: A Critique of Political Economy, Volume 1.* Trans. Ben Fowkes. London: Penguin Books.

Menon, Meera and Neera Adarkar (2005) *One Hundred Years, One Hundred Voices: The Mill Workers of Girangaon: An Oral History.* Bombay: Seagull.

Omvedt, Gail (1983) "Textile Strike Turns Political," *Economic and Political Weekly*, 27 August: 1511.

Petryna, Adriana (2005a) "Ethical Variability: Drug Development and Globalizing Clinical Trials," *American Ethnologist*, 32(2): 183–97.

Petryna, Adriana (2005b) "Drug Development and the Ethics of the Globalized Clinical Trial." Institute of Advanced Studies working paper.

Rabinow, Paul (1992) "Artificiality and Enlightenment: From Sociobiology to Biosociality," *Incorporations.* New York: Zone Books.

Rabinow, Paul (1996) *Essays on the Anthropology of Reason.* Princeton, NJ: Princeton University Press.

Rajagopal, Arvind (2004) "The Menace of Hawkers: Property Forms and the Politics of Liberalization in Mumbai" in Katherine Verdery and Caroline Humphrey (eds) *Property in Question: Value Transformation in the Global Economy.* New York: Berg.

Roy, Tirthankar (1993) *Artisans and Industrialization: Indian Weaving in the Twentieth Century.* Delhi: Oxford University Press.

Sassen, Saskia (2000) *Cities in a World Economy.* Thousand Oaks, CA: Pine Forge Press.

Spivak, Gayatri (1988) "Can the Subaltern Speak?" in C. Nelson and L. Grossberg (eds) *Marxism and the Interpretation of Culture.* Urbana and Chicago, IL: University of Illinois Press.

Spivak, Gayatri (1999) *A Critique of Postcolonial Reason: Toward a History of the Vanishing Present.* Cambridge, MA: Harvard University Press.

Sunder Rajan, Kaushik (2005) "Subjects of Speculation: Emergent Life Sciences and Market Logics in the US and India," *American Anthropologist*, 107(1): 19–30.

Sunder Rajan, Kaushik (2006) *Biocapital: The Constitution of Post-Genomic Life.* Durham, NC: Duke University Press.

Sunder Rajan, Rajeswari (1993) *Real and Imagined Women: Gender, Culture, and Postcolonialism.* New York and London: Routledge.

Trivedi, Harish (2003) "Cyber-coolies: Hindi and English," *Times Literary Supplement*, 27 June.

Tsing, Anna (2004) *Friction: An Ethnography of Global Connection.* Princeton, NJ: Princeton University Press.

Van Wersch, Hubert W.M. (1992) *The Bombay Textile Strike, 1982–83.* Bombay: Oxford University Press.

Williams, Raymond (1973) "Base and Superstructure in Marxist Cultural Theory," *New Left Review*, 82.

Afterword

Concept work

Paul Rabinow

I coined the term "biosociality" in the early 1990s at the very beginning of a research project on the human genome mapping initiative.[1] The term stood as a contrast to the then current term "socio-biology," a crude form of biological and evolutionary determinism. With the genome projects and the progress of molecular biology and related disciplines during the 1990s, socio-biology has passed from the scene to be replaced by a host of other world view projects purporting to reveal the deep meaning of evolution and of human existence. Additionally, the term "biosociality" was forged against the background of vivid scenes remembered from Thomas Mann's *The Magic Mountain*, scenes that moved me and seemed more pertinent to how disease, science, and fate were confronted than the thin narratives of socio-biology or its successors. I posed the question to myself: What had changed since the time when the self-quarantined, European bourgeoisie trudged the halls of its luxurious sanitariums with their X-rays under their arms, before and after sitting at sumptuous meals supplemented by diatribes on the meaning of Western civilization? While Mann filled his pages with disease ravaged bodies and tormented souls, clearly his real subject matter was a civilization whose health and pathology were in question and whose prognosis was poor. At the very least the geo-politics had changed and, more specifically, biology had changed. Of course, older forms of disease related sociality not focused on genes or molecules continue to this day. So, the question was: how had sociality changed given the rise of the new understanding of genetics? Thus, the term biosociality was coined as an initial attempt at framing the issues of a re-problematization of "life." Appropriately, the concept was an under-developed element in an initial orientation to what appeared to be an emergent domain of potential significance.

My approach was shaped by my previous work. I had recently completed *French Modern: Norms and Forms of the Social Environment*, a genealogical treatment of the social in France.[2] The book traced lines of emergence of a new object, "society" (and later "the social") that began to take shape in the cholera epidemics in the 1830s when the older medical nosology collapsed under the weight of events and effects that simply could not be captured or comprehended by the then current understandings of disease, of power relations, of spatial arrangements, and of meaning. Vital forces came bearing down, breaking open older configurations; consequently the need to address the existence of a space of problematization rapidly attained an urgency for which the powers that be were unprepared. What was going on? And what could be done about it?

French Modern showed that gradually, and in a disparate and temporally uneven manner, over the course of more than a century, a new object of power and knowledge had been formed in multiple foundries; work that required vast amounts of labor, especially as there was initially no blueprint available to decide what to assemble or precisely what directions to proceed in. The lack of a plan did not mean that an avalanche of proposals and convictions had not accrued, quite the contrary. That object was modern, i.e. it was produced in such a way that its knowledge component invited, even compelled, intervention and reform, a specific dynamic type of norming. The subset of "society" that was worked over in this manner was "the social."

One core lesson of the project was that the task of understanding the history of the present could be done following (and modifying) that peculiar genealogical history that Michel Foucault had wrought with such idiosyncratic brilliance. Today, it is clearer that the method is especially well-suited to configurations that are themselves, once again, being put into question and becoming a problem. That is to say, when the older configuration in the process of dis-aggregating under new pressures becomes more visible.

Casting about for a new project, French friends, students of Georges Canguilhem among others, suggested that I work on new figurations, concepts and practices of "life." They argued that there were significant aspects of the term's past that had been uncovered in *French Modern* (neo-Lamarckianism in France, public health, epidemic control, state population measures, and the like) and that new advances in molecular biology were plausibly contributing to a re-problematization of what were taken to be serious speech acts about living beings. After some reluctance and even amusement at the scale of the undertaking, I decided to take the proverbial plunge.

As with the term "society" (the social really didn't exist in the English speaking world), the challenge with seemingly universal terms – "but don't all societies have society?" – was to show how, at least to the degree that they were subject to truth claims, they were not universals but rather historical formations with distinctive elements following specific trajectories and subject to diverse contingent constraints, obscured by measures that erased or obliterated those specificities and contingencies. Thus, while presumably everyone would agree that the life sciences changed – that is what sciences were supposed to do after all – not everyone was comfortable with the idea that the referent of the life sciences had changed as well. It is both troubling and obvious that any scientific method must define, delimit, and work over its objects. And even those who were comfortable with that idea were not very clear about how best to describe this situation. This was the moment, we should remember, of the ascendancy in certain distinct university domains of the social studies of science and technology as well as that of its opponents both internal and external.

Term = word + concept + referent

Following John Dewey and Richard McKeon, we can define a "term" as a word plus a concept plus a referent. This internal distinction enables us to see more clearly how biosociality has operated, as well as something about its limits. The fifteen or so years that have elapsed after its coinage provide an opportunity to reflect on how a concept works in a field of uncoordinated inquiries.

Two or three aspects are immediately pertinent. When the term was coined in the early 1990s, it was an invented word linked to a preliminary formulation of a concept of how different domains of practice (genomics, pastoral care, patients' rights, alliances with researchers, etc.) might cohere in the future. In that sense one could say it operated in a space of virtuality and not potentiality. There was nothing pre-ordained waiting to be realized or fulfilled. Rather, still inchoate and vibrant forces began to be set in motion. Said another way, biosociality in the early 1990s was as much in search of a referent or space of reference as it was an act of naming such a domain that was already there. As Mann's novel, or the polio epidemic, or many other such instances indicate, there had been patient groups who had practiced a kind of sociality around a particular disease and it, vicissitudes, even ones with a genetic core (or presumed genetic core). But it was only with the human genome initiative and its mobilization of specific publics and interest groups of patients, physicians, and scientists around what Lily Kay has nicely called "a molecular vision of life" that a distinctive contemporary terrain began to be populated and given contour. The horizon of a new and comprehensive understanding of the gene and genetics became visible, or so it was plausible to believe. Hence when the concept was coined, it had a future orientation. In a soft sense, it was a prediction but more precisely it was an element in a broader analytic orientation. The concept seemed worth using in inquiry, testing in experience, observing in action, as the practices it sought to illuminate developed or withered, were contested and survived or thrived, met resistance and were blocked or overcame or skirted those attempting to thwart developments. Scientifically speaking there was no way to know beforehand what was going to happen.

During the 1990s, the domain of reference gradually filled out. This process was related directly to an accumulating corpus of data and knowledge: first, of the physical map of the human genome, then other maps; and, by the end of the decade a sequence, a rough draft of the Code of Codes, to mix several of the most prominent (and we now see as mis-guided) analogies of the decade. It may be that the 1990s will be seen as the Golden Age of Molecular Biosociality. There was hope, there was progress, there was a reason to be urgent even strident – there were reasons to want to be biosocial. Many works, chronicled in journalism, scholarly production, grant proposals, and laboratory note books, attest to the experiences, labors, sufferings, and moments of joy, of those involved. This period was a formative one when technology-driven advances in understanding were undeniable – a moment when it still seemed legitimate to have hope for dramatic, even definitive, diagnostic and therapeutic triumphs. Critics and skeptics certainly existed though much (but not all) of their criticism of genetic determinism was itself no more grounded in knowledge than were the hyperbolic claims of their opponents.

The initial use of the term "biosociality" was a heuristic one. And its utility was confirmed: referents were produced, practices invented, connections made, assemblages assembled, apparatuses put into motion. By the turn of the new century, however, some of the limits of the concept could now be seen with more clarity. The identification of such limitations is most welcome as biosociality was intended as a concept and not as an epochal designation meant to characterize an age or era, that is to say that by definition the term did not have the same analytic power everywhere. In some domains referents for the term proliferated, in others, apparently they never were produced at all. These limitations were a confirmation of the approach not its refutation. Inquiry reveals specificities and limits, an excellent definition of critical thinking.

Once the sequence of the human genome was established in a rough and ready fashion, the referent of the concept and perhaps some of its elements began to be put into question. For a start, both the "once we sequence the genome" hype and deflation were no longer timely. The genome was sequenced and it turned out there were only one quarter or so of the "genes" that were expected. This startling discovery has been downplayed by supporters and opponents alike, as well as among the leading scientists. It turns out, as Sydney Brenner, among others, has argued, that the advance of the sequencing projects revealed that the concept of the gene needed to be altered. Science progressed but at a different pace in different terms in different domains. The topology of the social and that of molecular biology are not the same. The redefinition of the gene and of genetic action shifted rapidly. A whole range of RNA activity that influenced how nucleic acids operated was discovered with surprising rapidity. New questions made possible by older progress opened new horizons.

As Talia Dan-Cohen and I chronicled in our account of the early years of Celera Diagnostics, *A Machine to Make a Future*, level-headed and well-informed scientists and business people invested large amounts of money drawn from a parent company on the idea that the basic genetic understanding of health and disease was still a plausible one.[3] Their emphasis was on diagnostics but as we observed there was a confidence in the company that the path to diagnostics was intertwined with the path to therapeutics. Gene action and variation would hold a key. The Celera Diagnostics' scientists, lawyers, and managers forged contractual arrangements with biosocially organized groups, formed together by a common pathology – Alzheimer's, breast cancer, asthma, etc. – who were eager for their condition to be specified at the molecular level and were pushing for Celera to devote its powerful resources at their condition. These groups provided either directly or indirectly through their connections with clinical institutions the large scale tissue samples and clinical records, Celera required to bring its project to fruition.

However, as several of the papers in this volume astutely demonstrate, things are changing. Taking the examples of Alzheimer's and autism, we observe a shifting of the time horizon. Former understandings of these terrible pathologies have to a degree re-appeared as the hopes and hype of the genomic decade have failed to provide adequate diagnostic or risk assessment tools or treatments based on them. Of course, hope and promises continue so that in a strict sense it makes no sense to claim that they can come true. But, we are rather more wary today than fifteen years ago. Hence a range of older understandings have resurfaced and with them a reconfigured terrain of meaning. The depth sought is not only in the future but also in futures past. And in presents to come.

Does biosociality still have any analytic power? It seems to me it does precisely because its contours of applicability, the specification of its elements, and the range of variations it covers are now clearer. Had the term ever been meant as an epochal term – which it never was – then it might well be time to toss it into the large dust bin of tropes, sweeping characterizations of "the age," and world views, for which there is an unending appetite. The term was not intended as a universal. It does not apply everywhere and at all times. However, there is a distinct gratification in watching emerge its more precise delimitations, its boundaries, and the extent of its dynamic range. Counter-events and other problematizations now appear more clearly as arenas of research.

We certainly need a broader range of concepts and more refinement in the ones we already have in our inventory. That being said, it is clear that neither the path of essentializing moves characteristic of an older anthropology – "not in my village" – nor those of newer cultural studies – "not in my civilization" – will provide them. Nor will simple empirical work do the job either. Advance requires conceptual elaboration and inquiry that is designed to be recursively critical. And that work will take place; it seems to me, increasingly in centers of sustained problem formation and inquiry such as the BIOS Center at the LSE or the Anthropology of the Contemporary Collaboratory (ARC) whose origins are in Berkeley.[4] But these are only beginnings; one looks forward with impatience to the proliferation of new forms of knowledge production and practice as problems globalize and as the older essentialisms become even more dated and thin than they are today.

Notes

1   Thanks for helpful comments to Mary Murrell, Stephen Collier, Tobias Rees, Marilyn Seid, Carlos Novas.
2   Paul Rabinow, *French Modern: Norms and Forms of the Social Environment*, Cambridge, MA: MIT Press, 1989; paperback, University of Chicago Press. French translation *Une France Si Moderne*, Paris: Buchet and Chastel, 2006.
3   Paul Rabinow and Talia Dan-Cohen, *A Machine to Make a Future: Biotech Chronicles*, Princeton, NJ: Princeton University Press, 2004; paperback with new Afterword, 2006.
4   Websites: www.anthropos-lab.net; www.lse.ac.uk/collections/BIOS/Default.htm.

Index